THE LARYNGECTOMEE GUIDE

Itzhak Brook, MD, MSc

TABLE OF CONTENTS

DEDICATION

The book is dedicated to my fellow laryngectomees and their caregivers for their courage and perseverance.

ACKNOWLEDGEMENT

I am grateful to Joyce Reback Brook and Carole Kaminsky for their editorial assistance.

DISCLAIMER

Dr Brook is not an expert in otolaryngology and head and neck surgery. This guide is not a substitute for medical care by medical professionals.

INTRODUCTION

I am a physician who became a laryngectomee in 2008. I was diagnosed with laryngeal cancer in 2006 and was initially treated with a course of radiation. After experiencing a recurrence two years later, my doctors recommended that total laryngectomy was the best assurance for eradicating the cancer. As I write this, it has been over five years since my operation; there has been no sign of recurrence.

After becoming a laryngectomee, I realized the magnitude of the challenges faced by new laryngectomees in learning how to care for themselves. Overcoming these challenges requires mastering new techniques in caring for one's airways, dealing with life long side effects of radiation and other treatments, living with the results of surgeries, facing uncertainties about the future, and struggling with psychological, social, medical and dental issues. I also learned the difficulties of life as a head and neck cancer survivor. This cancer and its treatment affect some of the most basic human functions, communication, nutrition, and social interaction.

As I gradually learned to cope with my life as a laryngectomee, I realized that the solutions to many problems are not only based on medicine and science but also on experience in addition to trial and error. I also realized that what works for one person may not always work for another. Because each person's medical history, anatomy and personality are different, so are some of the solutions. However, some general principles of care are helpful to most laryngectomees. I was fortunate to benefit from my physicians, speech and language pathologists, and other laryngetomees as I learned how to care for myself and overcome the myriad of daily challenges.

1

I gradually realized that new and even seasoned laryngectomees would probably improve their quality of life from learning how to better care for themselves. To that end I created a Website (http://dribrook.blogspot.com/) to help laryngectomees and other individuals with head and neck cancer. The site deals with medical, dental and psychological issues and also contains links to videos about rescue breathing and other informative lectures.

This practical guide is based on my Website and is aimed at providing useful information that can assist laryngectomees and their caregivers in dealing with medical, dental and psychological issues. The guide contains information about the side effects of radiation and chemotherapy; the methods of speaking after laryngectomy; how to care for the airway, stoma, heat and moisture exchange filter, and voice prosthesis. In addition I address eating and swallowing issues, medical, dental and psychological concerns, respiration and anesthesia, and travelling as a laryngectomee.

This guide is not a substitute for professional medical care but hopefully will be useful for laryngectomees and their caregiver(s) in dealing with their lives and the challenges they face.

CHAPTER 1:

Diagnosis and treatment of laryngeal cancer

Overview

Laryngeal cancer affects the voice box. Cancers that start in the larynx are called laryngeal cancers; cancers of the hypopharynx are called **hypopharyngeal cancers**. (The hypopharynx is the part of the throat [pharynx] that lies beside and behind the larynx.) These cancers are very close to each other and the treatment principles of both are similar and may involve laryngectomy. Although the discussion below addresses laryngeal cancer, it is also generally applicable to hypopharyngeal cancer.

Laryngeal cancer occurs when malignant cells appear in the larynx. The larynx contains the vocal cords (or folds) which, by vibrating, generate sounds that create audible voice when the vibrations echo through the throat, mouth, and nose.

The larynx is divided into three anatomical regions: the glottis (in the middle of the larynx, includes the vocal cords); the supraglottis (in the top part, includes the epiglottis, arytenoids and aryepiglottic folds, and false cords); and the subglottis (the bottom of the larynx). While cancer can develop in any part of the larynx most laryngeal cancers originate in the glottis. Supraglottic cancers are less common, and subglottic tumors are the least frequent.

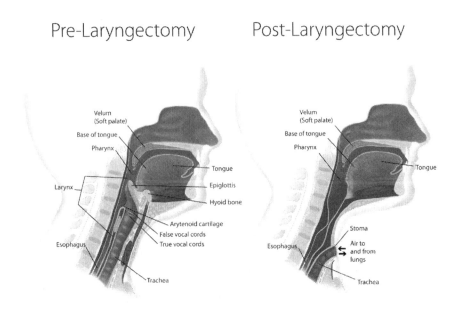

Figure 1: Anatomy before and after laryngectomy

Laryngeal and hypopharyngeal cancer may spread by direct extension to adjacent structures, by metastasis to regional cervical lymph nodes, or more distantly, through the blood stream to other locations in the body. Distant metastases to the lungs and liver are most common. Squamous cell carcinomas account for 90 to 95 percent of laryngeal and hypopharyngeal cancer.

Smoking and heavy alcohol consumption are the main risk factors for laryngeal cancer. Exposure to human papilloma virus (HPV) has been mainly associated with oropharyngeal cancer and to a lesser degree with laryngeal and hypopharyngeal ones.

There are about 50,000 to 60,000 laryngectomees in the USA. According to the Surveillance Epidemiology and End Results (SEER) Cancer Statistics Review of the National Cancer Institute, an estimated 12,250 men and women are diagnosed with cancer of the larynx each year. The number of new laryngectomees has been declining mainly because fewer people are smoking and newer therapeutic approaches can spare the larynx.

Diagnosis

Symptoms and signs of laryngeal cancer include:

- Abnormal (high-pitched) breathing sounds

- Chronic cough (with and without blood)

- Difficulty swallowing

- A sensation of a lump in the throat

- Hoarseness that does not get better in 1 - 2 weeks

- Neck and ear pain

- Sore throat that does not get better in 1 - 2 weeks, even with antibiotics

- Swelling or lumps in the neck

- Unintentional weight loss

The symptoms associated with laryngeal cancer depend upon its location. Persistent hoarseness can be the initial complaint in cancers of the glottis. Later symptoms may include difficulty in swallowing, ear pain, chronic and sometimes bloody cough, and hoarseness. Supraglottic cancers are frequently diagnosed only when they cause airway obstruction or palpable metastatic lymph nodes. Primary subglottic tumors typically present with hoarseness or complaints of difficulty in breathing on exertion.

There is no single test that can accurately diagnose cancer. The complete evaluation of a patient generally requires a thorough history and physical examination along with diagnostic testing. Many tests are required to determine if a person has cancer or if another condition (such as an infection) may be mimicking the symptoms of cancer.

Effective diagnostic testing is used to confirm or eliminate the presence of cancer, monitor its progress, and plan for and evaluate the effectiveness of treatment. In some instances, it is necessary to perform repeat testing if a person's condition has changed, a sample collected was not of good quality, or an abnormal test result needs to be confirmed. Diagnostic procedures for cancer may include imaging, laboratory tests, tumor biopsy, endoscopic examination, surgery, or genetic testing.

The following tests and procedures may be used to help diagnose and stage laryngeal cancer which influences the choice of treatment:

Physical examination of the throat and neck: This enables the doctor to feel for swollen lymph nodes in the neck and to view the throat by using a small, long-handled mirror to check for abnormalities.

Endoscopy: A procedure in which an endoscope (a flexible lighted tube) is inserted through the nose or mouth into the upper airway to the larynx, enabling the examiner to directly view these structures.

Laryngoscopy: A procedure to examine the larynx with a mirror or a laryngoscope (a rigid lighted tube).

CT scan (computed tomography): A procedure that generates a series of detailed radiographs of body sites, taken from different directions. A contrast material such as an injected or swollen dye enables better visualization of the organs or tissues.

MRI (magnetic resonance imaging): A procedure that uses a magnet and radio waves to generate a series of detailed pictures of areas inside the body.

Barium swallow: A procedure to examine the esophagus and stomach in which the patient drinks a barium solution that coats the esophagus and stomach, and x-rays are obtained.

Biopsy: A procedure in which tissues are obtained so that they can be viewed under a microscope to check for cancer.

The potential for recovery from laryngeal cancer depends on the following:

- The extent the cancer has spread (the "stage")

- The appearance of the cancer cells (the "grade")

- The location(s) and size of the tumor

- The patient's age, gender, and general health

Additionally, smoking tobacco and drinking alcohol decrease the effectiveness of treatment for laryngeal cancer. Patients with laryngeal cancer who continue to smoke and drink are less likely to be cured and more likely to develop a second tumor.

Treatment of laryngeal cancer

Individuals with early or small laryngeal cancer may be treated with surgery or radiation therapy. Those with advanced laryngeal cancer may require a combination of treatments. This may include surgery and a combination of radiation therapy and chemotherapy, generally given at the same time.

Targeted therapy is another therapeutic option specifically directed at advanced laryngeal cancer. Targeted cancer therapies are administered by using drugs or other substances that block the growth and spread of cancer by interfering with specific molecules involved in tumor growth and progression.

The choice of treatment depends mainly on the patient's general health, the location of the tumor, and whether the cancer has spread to other sites.

A team of medical specialists generally collaborate in planning the treatment.

These can include:

- Ear, nose, and throat doctors (otolaryngologists)

- General head and neck surgeons

- Medical oncologists

- Radiation oncologists

Other health care providers who work with the specialists as a team may include a dentist, plastic surgeon, reconstructive surgeon, speech and language pathologist, oncology nurse, dietitian, and a mental health counselor.

Treatment options depend on the following:

- The extent to which the cancer has spread (the "stage")

- The location and size of the tumor

- Maintaining the patient's ability to talk, eat, and breathe as normally as possible

- Whether the cancer has returned

The medical team describes the available treatment choices to the patient and what are the expected results, as well as the possible side effects. Patients should carefully consider the available options and understand how these treatments may affect their ability to eat, swallow, and talk, and whether these treatments will alter their appearance during and after treatment. The patient and his/her health care team can work together to develop a treatment plan that fits the patient's needs and expectations.

Supportive care for control of pain and other symptoms that can relieve potential side effects and ease emotional concerns should be available before, during, and after cancer treatment.

Patients should be well informed before making their choice. If necessary, obtaining a second medical and/or surgical opinion is helpful. Having a patient advocate (family member or friend) attend the discussions with the medical team is desirable as they can assist the patient in making the best choice.

It is suggested to ask the following questions of the medical team:

- What is the size, location, spread, and stage of the tumor?

- What are the treatment options? Would they include surgery, radiation therapy, chemotherapy or a combination of these?

- What are the expected side effects, risks and benefits of each kind of treatment?

- How can side effects be managed?

- What will be the sound of the voice with each of the above treatments?

- What are the chances of being able to eat normally?

- How to prepare for treatment?

- Will the treatment require hospitalization and if so for how long?

- What is the estimated cost of the treatment and will insurance cover it?

- How will the treatment affect one's life, work and normal activities?

- Is a research study (clinical trial) a good option?

- Can the physician recommend an expert for a second opinion regarding the treatment options?

- How often and for how long will there be a need for follow-ups?

CHAPTER 2:

Having surgery: types of laryngectomy, outcome, pain management, and seeking a second opinion

Types of laryngectomy

Treatment of laryngeal cancer often includes surgery. The surgeon can use either scalpel or laser. Laser surgery is performed using a device that generates an intense beam of light that cuts or destroys tissues.

There are two types of surgery for removal of laryngeal cancer:

Removal of part of the larynx: The surgeon takes out only the part of the larynx harboring the tumor.

Removal of the entire larynx: The surgeon removes the whole larynx and some adjacent tissues.

Lymph nodes that are close or drain the cancerous site may also be taken out during either type of surgery.

The patient may need to undergo reconstructive or plastic surgery to rebuild the affected tissues. The surgeon may obtain tissues from other parts of the body to repair the site of the surgery in the throat and/ or neck. The reconstructive or plastic surgery sometimes takes place at the same time when the cancer is removed, or it can be performed later.

Healing after surgery takes time; the length of time needed to recover varies among individuals.

Surgery's outcome

The main results of the surgery can include all or some of the following:

- Throat and neck swelling

- Local pain

- Tiredness

- Increased mucus production

- Changes in physical appearance

- Numbness, muscle stiffness and weakness

- Tracheostomy

Most people feel weak or tired for some time after surgery, have a swollen neck, and experience pain and discomfort for the first few days. Pain medications can relieve some of these symptoms. (See **Pain management,** page 101)

Surgery can alter the ability to swallow, eat, or talk. However, not all such effects are permanent, as discussed later in the guide (see chapters 6 and 11). Those who lose their ability to talk after surgery may find it useful to communicate by writing on a notepad, writing board (such as a magic slate), cell phone, or computer. Prior to the surgery it may be helpful to make a recording for one's answering machine or voicemail to inform callers about one's speaking difficulties.

An electrolarynx can be used to speak within a few days after the surgery. (See **Electrolarynx,** page 47) Because of neck swelling and post surgical stitches the intra-oral route of delivering vibrations with a straw-like tube is preferred.

Preparing for surgery

Prior to surgery it is important to thoroughly discuss with the surgeon all available therapeutic and surgical options and their short and long term outcomes. Patients scheduled for surgery may be anxious and under a lot of stress. It is therefore important to have a patient advocate (such as a family member or friend) also attend the meetings with the surgeon. It is important to freely ask and discuss any concerns and request clarifications. It may be necessary to repeatedly listen to explanations until they are fully understood. It is useful to prepare questions to ask the surgeon prior to the meeting and write down the information obtained.

In addition to consultation with the surgeon, it is also important to see these medical providers:

- Internist and/or family physician

- Any specialist one sees for a specific medical problem (i.e., cardiologist, pulmonologist, etc.)

- Radiation oncologist

- Medical oncologist

- Anesthetist

- Dentist

- Speech and language pathologist (SLP)

- Social worker or mental health counselor

- Nutritionist

It is also very useful to meet other individuals who have already undergone a laryngectomy. They can guide the patient about future speech options, share some of their experiences, and provide emotional support.

Getting a second opinion

When facing a new medical diagnosis that requires making a choice between several therapeutic options, including surgery, it is important to get a second opinion. There may be different medical and surgical approaches and a second (or even third) opinion may be invaluable. Getting such an opinion from physicians experienced in the issues at hand is judicious. There are many situations when treatment cannot be reversed. This is why choosing the course of therapy after consulting with at least one more specialist is very important.

Some individuals may be reluctant to ask for a referral to see another physician for a second opinion. Some may be afraid that this will be interpreted as lack of confidence in their primary physician or doubts about their competence. Most physicians encourage their patients to get a second opinion and will not feel insulted or intimidated by such a request. Furthermore, many medical insurers welcome it.

The second doctor may agree with the first doctor's diagnosis and treatment plan. Conversely, the other physician may suggest a different approach. Either way, the patient ends up with more valuable information and also with a greater sense of control. Eventually one may feel more confident about the decisions he/she makes, knowing that all options have been considered.

Gathering one's medical records and seeing another physician may take some time and effort. Generally, the delay in initiating treatment will not make the eventual treatment less effective. However, one should discuss any possible delay with the physician.

There are numerous ways to find an expert for a second opinion. One can request a referral to another specialist from the primary doctor, a local or state medical society, a nearby hospital, or a medical school. Even though patients with cancer are often in a rush to get treated and remove the cancer as soon as possible, waiting for another opinion may be worthwhile.

Pain management after surgery

The degree of pain experienced after laryngecomy (or any other head and neck surgery) is very subjective, but, as a general rule, the more extensive the surgery, the more likely the patient will experience pain. Certain types of reconstructive procedures, where tissue is transferred (a flap) from the chest muscles, forearm, thigh, jejunum, or a stomach pull up are more likely to be associated with increased or prolonged pain.

Those who have a radical neck dissection as part of the surgery may experience additional pain. At present, most patients undergo a "modified radical neck dissection" when the spinal accessory nerve is not removed. If the spinal accessory nerve is cut or removed during surgery, the patient is more likely to have shoulder discomfort, stiffness, and long term loss of range of motion. Some of the attendant discomfort of this procedure can be prevented by exercise and physical therapy.

For individuals who experience chronic pain as a result of laryngectomy or any other head and neck surgery, evaluation by a pain management specialist is usually very helpful. (See **Pain management, page 101**)

CHAPTER 3:

Side effects of radiation treatment for head and neck cancer

Radiation therapy (RT) is often used to treat head and neck cancer. The goal of RT is to kill cancer cells. Because these cells divide and grow at a faster rate than normal cells, they are more likely to be destroyed by radiation. In contrast, although they may be damaged healthy cells generally recover.

If RT is recommended the radiation oncologist sets up a treatment plan that includes the total dose of radiation to be administered, the number of treatments to be given, and their schedule. These are based on the type and location of the tumor, the patient's general health, and other present or past treatments.

The side effects of RT for head and neck cancer are divided into early (acute) and long term (chronic). Early side effects occur during the course of therapy and during the immediate post therapy period (approximately 2-3 weeks after the completion of a course of RT). Chronic effects can manifest any time thereafter, from weeks to years later.

Patients are usually most bothered by the early effects of RT, although these will generally resolve over time. However, because long term effects may require lifelong care it is important to recognize these in order to prevent them and/or deal with their consequences. Knowledge of the radiation side effects can allow their early detection and proper management.

Individuals with head and neck cancer should receive counseling about the importance of smoking cessation. In addition to the fact that smoking is a major risk factor for head and neck cancer, the risk of cancer in smokers is further enhanced by alcohol consumption. Smoking can also influence cancer prognosis. When smoking is continued both during and after RT, it can increase the severity and duration of mucosal reactions, worsen the dry mouth (xerostomia), and compromise patient outcome. Patients who continue to smoke while receiving RT have a lower long-term survival rate than those who do not smoke. (See **Avoiding smoking and alcohol,** page 115)

1. Early side effects

Early side effects include inflammation of the oropharyngeal mucosa (mucositis), painful swallowing (odynophagia), difficulty swallowing (dysphagia), hoarseness, lack of saliva (xerostomia), orofacial pain, dermatitis, nausea, vomiting, and weight loss. These complications can interfere with, and delay treatment. To some degree, these side effects occur in most patients and generally dissipate over time.

The severity of these side effects is influenced by the amount and method by which the RT is given, the tumor's location and spread, and the patient's general health and habits (i.e., continued smoking, alcohol consumption).

Skin damage

Radiation can cause a sunburn-like damage to the skin which can be further aggravated by chemotherapy. It is advisable to avoid exposure to potential chemical irritants, direct sun and wind, and local application of lotions or ointments prior to RT that might change the depth of radiation penetration. There are a number of skin care products that can be used during radiation treatment to lubricate and protect the skin.

Dry mouth

The loss of saliva production (or xerostomia) is related to the administered irradiation dose and the volume of salivary tissue irradiated. Drinking adequate fluids and rinsing and gargling with a weak solution of salt and baking soda are helpful to refresh the mouth, loosen thick oral secretions, and alleviate mild pain. Artificial saliva and constant wetting of the mouth with water may also be helpful.

Alterations in taste

Radiation can induce changes in taste as well as tongue pain. Such side effects can further decrease food intake. The altered taste and tongue pain gradually dissipate in most patients over a six month period, although in some cases taste recovery is incomplete. Many individuals experience a permanent alteration in their taste.

Inflammation of the oropharyngeal mucosa (mucositis)

Radiation, as well as chemotherapy, damage the oropharyngeal mucosa, resulting in mucositis which develops gradually, usually two to three weeks after starting RT. Its incidence and severity depend upon the field, total dose and duration of RT. Chemotherapy can aggravate the condition. Mucositis can be painful and interfere with food intake and nutrition.

Management includes meticulous oral hygiene, dietary modification, and topical anesthetics combined with an antacid and antifungal suspension ("cocktail"). Spicy, acidic, sharp, or hot food should be avoided, as well as all alcohol. Secondary bacterial, viral (e.g., Herpes), and fungal (e.g., Candida) infections are possible. Control of the pain (using opiates or gabapentin) may be needed.

Mucositis can lead to nutritional deficiency. Those who experience significant weight loss or recurrent episodes of dehydration may require feeding through a gastrostomy feeding tube.

Orofacial pain

Orofacial pain is common in patients with head and neck cancer and occurs in up to half of the patients before RT, eighty percent of patients during treatment and about one third of patients six months after treatment. The pain can be caused by mucositis which can be aggravated by concurrent chemotherapy, and by damage from the cancer, infection, inflammation, and scarring due to surgery or other treatments. Pain management includes the use of analgesics and narcotics. (See **Pain management,** page 101).

Nausea and vomiting

RT may cause nausea. When it occurs, it generally happens from two to six hours after a RT session and generally lasts about two hours. Nausea may or may not be accompanied by vomiting.

Management includes:

- Eating small, frequent meals throughout the day instead of three large meals. Nausea is often worse if the stomach is empty.

- Eating slowly, chewing the food completely, and staying relaxed.

- Eating cold or room temperature foods. The smell of hot or warm foods may induce nausea.

- Avoiding difficult to digest foods, such as spicy foods or foods high in fat or accompanied by rich sauces.

- Resting after eating. When lying down, the head should be elevated about 12 inches.

- Drinking beverages and other fluids between meals instead of drinking beverages with meals.

- Drinking 6- 8 ounce glasses of fluid per day to prevent dehydration. Cold beverages, ice cubes, popsicles, or gelatin are adequate.

- Eating more food at a time of the day when one is less nauseous.

- Informing one's health care provider before each treatment session when one develops persistent nausea.

- Treating persistent vomiting immediately, as this can cause dehydration.

- Administering anti-nausea medication by a health care provider.

Persistent vomiting can result in the body losing large amounts of water and nutrients. If vomiting persists for more than three times a day and one does not drink enough fluids, it could lead to dehydration. This condition can cause serious complications if left untreated.

Signs of dehydration include:

- Small amount of urine

- Dark urine

- Rapid heart rate

- Headaches

- Flushed, dry skin

- Coated tongue

- Irritability and confusion

Persistent vomiting may reduce the effectiveness of medications. If persistent vomiting continues, RT may be stopped temporarily. Fluids administered intravenously assist the body in regaining nutrients and electrolytes.

Tiredness (fatigue)

Fatigue is one of the most common side effects of RT. RT can cause cumulative fatigue (fatigue that increases over time). It usually lasts from three to four weeks after treatment stops, but can continue for up to two to three months.

Factors that contribute to fatigue are anemia, decrease food and liquid intake, medications, hypothyroidism, pain, stress, depression, and lack of sleep (insomnia) and rest.

Rest, energy conservation, and correcting the above contributing factors may ameliorate the fatigue.

Other side effects

These include trismus (See page 24) and hearing problems (See page 27).

2. Late side effects

Late side effects of RT include permanent loss of saliva, osteoradionecrosis, ototoxicity, fibrosis, lymphedema, hypothyroidism, and damage to neck structures.

Permanent mouth dryness

Although dry mouth (xerostomia) improves in most people with time, it can be long lasting.

Management includes salivary substitutes or artificial saliva and frequent sips of water. This may lead to frequent urination during the night, especially in men with prostatic hypertrophy and in those with small bladders. Available treatment includes medications such as salivary stimulants (sialagogues), pilocarpine, amifostine, cevimeline, and acupuncture.

Osteoradionecrosis of the jaw

This is one potentially severe complication that may necessitate surgical intervention and reconstruction. Depending on the location and extent of the lesion, symptoms can include pain, bad breath, taste distortion (dysgeusia), "bad sensation", numbness (anesthesia), trismus, difficulty with mastication and speech, fistula formation, pathologic fracture, and local, spreading, or systemic infection.

The jaw bone (mandible) is the most frequently affected bone, especially in those treated for nasopharyngeal cancer. Maxillary involvement is rare because of the collateral blood circulation it receives.

Tooth extraction and dental disease in irradiated areas are major factors in the development of osteoradionecrosis. (See **Dental issues**, page 117) In some cases it is necessary to remove teeth before RT if they will be in the area receiving radiation and are too decayed to preserve by filling or root canal. An unhealthy tooth can serve as a source of infection to the jawbone, that can be particularly difficult to treat after radiation.

Repair of nonrestorable and diseased teeth prior to RT may reduce the risk of this complication. Mild osteoradionecrosis can be conservatively treated with debridement, antibiotics, and occasionally ultrasound. When necrosis is extensive, radical resection, followed by microvascular reconstruction, is often used.

Dental prophylaxis can reduce this problem. (See **Dental issues, page 117**) Special fluoride treatments may help with dental problems, along with brushing, flossing, and regular cleaning by a dental hygienist.

Hyperbaric oxygen therapy (HBO) has been often used in patients at risk or those who develop osteoradionecrosis of the jaw. However, the available data are conflicting about the clinical benefits of HBO for prevention and therapy of osteoradionecrosis. (See **Heperbaric oxygen therapy,** page 119)

Patients should remind their dentists about their RT prior to extraction or dental surgery. Osteoradionecrosis may be prevented by administration of a series of HBO therapy before and after these procedures. This is recommended if the involved tooth is in an area that has been exposed to a high dose of radiation. Consulting the radiation oncologist who delivered the radiation treatment can be helpful in determining the extent of prior exposure.

Fibrosis and trismus

High doses of radiation to the head and neck can result in fibrosis. This condition may be aggravated after head and neck surgery where the neck may develop a woody texture and have limited movement. Late onset of fibrosis can also occur in the pharynx and esophagus leading to stricture, and temporomandibular joint problems.

Fibrosis of the muscles of mastication can lead to the inability to open the mouth (**trismus or lockjaw**), which can progress over time. Generally, eating becomes more difficult but articulation is not affected. Trismus impedes proper oral care and treatment and may cause speech/swallowing deficits. This condition may be intensified by surgery prior to radiation. Patients likely to develop trismus are those with tumors of the nasopharynx, palate, and maxillary sinus. Radiation of the highly vascularized temporomandibular joint (TMJ) and muscles of mastication can often lead to trismus. Chronic trismus gradually leads to fibrosis. Trismus impedes proper oral care and treatment and may cause speech/swallowing deficits. Forced opening of the mouth, jaw exercises and the use of a dynamic opening device (Therabite™) can be helpful. This device is increasingly used during radiation therapy as a prophylactic measure to prevent trismus.

Exercise can reduce neck tightness and increases the range of neck motion. One needs to perform these exercises throughout life to maintain good neck mobility. This is especially the case if the stiffness is due to radiation. Receiving treatment by experienced physical therapies who can also break down the fibrosis is very helpful. The earlier the intervention, the better it is for the patient. A new treatment modality using external laser is also available. There are physical therapy experts in most communities who specialize in reducing swelling.

Fibrosis in the head and neck can become even more extensive in those who have surgery or further radiation. Post radiation fibrosis can also involve the skin and subcutanous tissues, causing discomfort and lymphedema.

Swallowing dysfunction due to fibrosis often requires a change in diet, pharyngeal strengthening, or swallow retraining especially in those who have had surgery and/or chemotherapy. Swallowing exercises are increasingly used as a preventing measure. (See Swallowing difficulties, page 91) Partial or total oropharyngeal stricture can occur in severe cases.

Wound healing problems

Some laryngectomees may manifest wound healing problems following surgery, especially in areas that have received RT. Some may develop a fistula (an abnormal connection between the inside of the throat and the skin). Wounds that heal at a slower pace can be treated with antibiotics and dressing changes. (See **Pharyngo-cutaneoius fistula,** page 98)

Lymphedema

Obstruction of the cutaneous lymphatics results in lymphedema. Significant pharyngeal or laryngeal edema may interfere with breathing and may require temporary or long term tracheostomy. Lymphedema, strictures, and other dysfunctions predispose patients to aspiration and the need for a feeding tube. (See **Lymphedema,** page 37).

Hypothyroidism

RT is almost always associated with hypothyroidism. The incidence varies; it is dose-dependent and increases with time since the RT. (See **Low thyroid hormone and its treatment,** page 105)

Neurological damage

RT to the neck can also affect the spinal cord, resulting in a self-limited transverse myelitis, known as "Lhermitte sign". The patient notes an electric shock-like sensation mostly felt with neck bending (flexion). This condition rarely progresses to a true transverse myelitis which is associated with Brown-Séquard syndrome (A loss of sensation and motor function caused by the lateral cutting of the spinal cord).

RT can also cause peripheral nervous system dysfunction resulting from external compressive fibrosis of soft tissues and reduced blood supply caused by fibrosis. Pain, sensory loss, and weakness are the most commonly observed clinical features of peripheral nervous system dysfunction. Autonomic dysfunction with resultant orthostatic hypotension (an abnormal decrease in blood pressure when a person stands up) and other abnormalities can also be seen.

Damage to the ear (ototoxicity)

Radiation to the ear may result in serous otitis (otitis with effusion). High doses of irradiation can cause and sensorineural hearing loss (damage to the inner ear, the auditory nerve, or the brain).

Damage to neck structures

Neck edema and fibrosis are common after RT. Over time the edema may harden, leading to neck stiffness. Damage can also include carotid artery narrowing (stenosis) and stroke, carotid artery rupture, oropharyngo-cutaneous fistula (the last two are associated also with surgery), and carotid artery baroreceptors damage leading to permanent and proxysmal (sudden and recurrent) hypertension.

Carotid artery narrowing (stenosis): The carotid arteries in the neck supply blood to the brain. Radiation to the neck has been linked to carotid artery stenosis or narrowing, representing a significant risk for head and neck cancer patients, including many laryngectomees. Stenosis can be diagnosed by ultrasound as well as angiography. It is important to diagnose carotid stenosis early, before a stroke has occurred.

Treatment includes removal of the blockage (endarterectomy), placing a stent (a small device placed inside the artery to widens it) or a prosthetic carotid bypass grafting.

Hypertension due to baroreceptors damage: Radiation to the head and neck can damage the baroreceptors located in the carotid artery. These baroreceptors (blood pressure sensors) help in regulating blood pressure by detecting the pressure of blood flowing through them, and sending messages to the central nervous system to increase or decrease the peripheral vascular resistance and cardiac output. Some individual treated with radiation develop labile or paroxysmal hypertension.

> **Labile hypertension:** In this condition the blood pressure fluctuates far more than usual during the day. It can rapidly soar from low (e.g.,120/80 mm Hg) to high (e.g., 170/105 mm Hg). In many instances these fluctuations are asymptomatic but may be associated with headaches. A relationship between blood pressure elevation and stress or emotional distress is usually present.

> **Paroxysmal hypertension:** Patients exhibit sudden elevation of blood pressure (which can be greater than 200/110 mm Hg) associated with an abrupt onset of distressful physical symptoms, such as headache, chest pain, dizziness, nausea, palpitations, flushing, and sweating. Episodes can last from 10 minutes to several hours and may occur once every few months to once or twice daily. Between episodes, the blood pressure is normal or may be mildly elevated. Patients generally cannot identify obvious psychological factors that cause the paroxysms. Medical conditions that can also cause such blood pressure swings need to be excluded (e.g., pheochromocytoma).

Both of these conditions are serious and should be treated. Management can be difficult and should be done by experienced specialists.

More information about complications of RT can be found at the National Cancer Institute Web site at:

http://www.cancer.gov/cancertopics/pdq/supportivecare/oralcomplications/Patient/page5

CHAPTER 4:

Side effects of chemotherapy for head and neck cancer

Chemotherapy for head and neck cancer is used in conjunction with supportive care for most patients with metastatic or advanced recurrent head and neck cancer. The choice of specific systemic therapy is influenced by the patient's prior treatment with chemotherapeutic agents and the general approach to preserve the effected organs. Supportive care includes the prevention of infection due to severe bone marrow suppression and the maintenance of adequate nutrition.

Therapeutic options include treatment with a single agent and combination regimens with conventional cytotoxic chemotherapy and/or molecularly targeted agents, combined with optimal supportive care. Chemotherapy is given in cycles, alternating between periods of treatment and rest. Treatment can last several months, or even longer.

A Web site that lists all the chemotherapeutic agents and their side effects is at: http://www.tirgan.com/chemolst.htm

Chemotherapeutic drugs which are usually given intravenously, work throughout the whole body by disrupting cancer cells' growth. Chemotherapy for the treatment of head and neck cancers is usually given at the same time as radiation therapy and is known as chemoradiation. It can be given as adjuvant chemotherapy or as neoadjuvant chemotherapy.

Adjuvant chemotherapy is used for treatment after surgery to reduce the risk of cancer returning, and to kill cells that may have spread. Neoadjuvant chemotherapy is administered before surgery to shrink the size of the tumor thus making it easier to remove.

Chemotherapy administered prior to chemoradiation treatment is known as induction chemotherapy.

Side effects of chemotherapy

The kind and type of possible side effects of chemotherapy depend on the individual. Some have few side effects, while others have more. Many individuals do not experience side effects until the end of their treatments; for many individuals these side effects do not last long.

Chemotherapy can, however, cause several temporary side effects. Although these may be worse with combined radiation therapy, they generally disappear gradually after the treatment has ended.

Side effects depend on the chemotherapeutic agent(s) used. These occur because chemotherapy drugs work by killing all actively growing cells. These include cells of the digestive tract, hair follicles, and bone marrow (which makes red and white blood cells), as well as the cancer cells.

The more common side effects are nausea, vomiting, diarrhea, sores (mucositis) in the mouth (resulting in problems with swallowing and sensitivity in the mouth and throat), increased susceptibility to infection, anemia, hair loss, general fatigue, numbness in the hands and feet, hearing loss, kidney damage, bleeding problems, malaise, and balance problem. An oncologist and other medical specialist watch for and treat these side effects.

The most common side effects include:

Lowered resistance to infection

Chemotherapy can temporarily reduce the production of white blood cells (neutropenia), making the patient more susceptible to infections.

This effect may begin about seven days following treatment and the decline in resistance to infection is maximal usually about 10–14 days after chemotherapy has ended. At that point the blood cells generally begin to increase steadily and return to normal before the next cycle of chemotherapy is administered. Signs of infection include fever above 100.4°F (38°C) and/or sudden feeling of being ill. Prior to resuming chemotherapy blood test are performed to ensure that the recovery of the white blood cells has occurred. Further administration of chemotherapy may be delayed until recovery of blood cells has taken place.

Bruising or bleeding

Chemotherapy can promote bruising or bleeding because the agents given reduce the production of platelets which help the blood clotting. Nosebleeds, blood spots or rashes on the skin, and bleeding gums can be a sign that this had occurred.

Anemia

Chemotherapy can lead to anemia (low number of red blood cells). The patient generally feels tired and breathless. Severe anemia can be treated by blood transfusions or medications that promote red cells production.

Hair loss

Some chemotherapy agents cause hair loss. The hair almost always grows back over a period of 3-6 months once the chemotherapy has ended. Meanwhile, a wig, bandana, hat or scarf can be worn.

Sore mouth and small mouth ulcers

Some chemotherapy agents cause sore mouth (mucositis) which can interfere with mastication and swallowing, oral bleeding, difficulty in swallowing (dysphagia), dehydration, heartburn, vomiting, nausea, and sensitivity to salty, spicy, and hot/cold foods. These agents can also cause chemotherapy-related oral cavity ulcers (stomatitis) that result in eating difficulty.

Nausea and vomiting can be treated by anti-nausea (anti-emetic) drugs. Regular mouthwashes can also help. These side effects can impact swallowing and nutrition. Accordingly, it is important to supplement one's diet with nutritious drinks or soups. A dietitian's advice may be helpful to maintain adequate nutrition.

The cytotoxic agents most often associated with oral, pharyngeal, and esophageal symptoms of swallowing difficulty (dysphagia) are the antimetabolites such as methotrexate and fluorouracil. The radiosensitizer chemotherapies, designed to heighten the effects of radiation therapy, also increase the side effects of the radiation mucositis.

Tiredness (fatigue)

Chemotherapy affects different individuals in different ways. Some people are able to lead a normal life during their treatment, while others may find they become very weak and tired (fatigue) and have to take things more slowly. Any chemotherapy drug may cause fatigue.

It can last for a few days or persists through and beyond completion of treatment. Drugs such as vincristine, vinblastine, and cisplatin often cause fatigue.

Factors that contribute to fatigue are anemia, decrease food and liquid intake, medications, hypothyroidism, pain, stress, depression, and lack of sleep (insomnia) and rest.

Rest, energy conservation, and correcting the above contributing factors may ameliorate the fatigue.

More information can be found at the National Cancer Institute Web site at:

http://www.cancer.gov/cancertopics/pdq/supportivecare/ oralcomplications/Patient/page5

CHAPTER 5:

Lymphedema, neck swelling and numbness after radiation and surgery

Lymphedema

The lymph vessels drain fluid from tissues throughout the body and allow immune cells to travel throughout the body. Lymphedema is a localized lymphatic fluid retention and tissue swelling caused by a compromised lymphatic system. Lymphedema, a common complication of radiation and surgery for head and neck cancer, is an abnormal accumulation of protein-rich fluid in the space between cells which causes chronic inflammation and reactive fibrosis of the affected tissues.

Radiation creates scarring which interferes with the function of the lymphatics. The cervical lymph nodes are generally removed when the cancer is excised. When the surgeons remove these glands, they also take away the drainage system for the lymphatics and cut some of the sensory nerves. Unfortunately, most of the severed lymphatics and nerves are permanently cut. Consequently it takes longer to drain the area, resulting in swelling. Like flooding after a heavy rain when the drainage system is broken, the surgery creates a backup of lymphatic fluid that cannot drain adequately, as well as numbness of the areas supplied by the severed nerves (usually in the neck, chin, and behind the ears). As a result, some of the lymphatic fluid cannot re-enter the systemic circulation and accumulates in the tissues.

There are two types of lymphedema that can develop in patients with head and neck cancer: an *external* visible swelling of the skin or soft tissue and an *internal* swelling of the mucosa of the pharynx and larynx. Lymphedema generally starts slowly and is progressive, rarely painful, causes discomfort in the form of a sensation of heaviness and achiness, and may lead to skin changes.

Lymphedema has several stages:

Stage 0: Latency stage – No visible/palpable edema

Stage 1: Accumulation of protein-rich edema, presence of pitting edema that can be reduced with elevation

Stage 2: Progressive pitting, proliferation of connective tissue (fibrosis)

Stage 3: No pitting, presence of fibrosis, sclerosis, and skin changes

Lymphedema of the head and neck can cause several functional impairments.

These include:

- Difficulty in breathing

- Impairment in vision

- Motor limitations (reduced neck motion, jaw tightness or trismus and chest tightness)

- Sensory limitations

- Speech, voice and swallowing problems (inability to use an electrolarynx, difficulty in articulation, drooling, and loss of food from mouth)

- Emotional issues (depression, frustration and embarrassment)

Fortunately over time the lymphatics find new ways of drainage and the swelling generally goes down. Specialists in reducing edema (usually physical therapists) can assist the patient in enhancing the drainage and shortening the time for the swelling to decrease. This intervention can also prevent the area from becoming permanently swollen and from developing fibrosis.

Treatment of lymphedema includes:

- Manual lymph drainage (face and neck, deep lymphatics, trunk, intra oral)

- Compressive bandages and garments

- Remedial exercises

- Skin care

- Elastic therapeutic tape (Kinesiotape)

- Oncology rehabilitation

- Diuretics, surgical removal (debulking), liposuction, compression pumps, and elevation of the head alone are ineffective treatments.

Neck tightness and swelling due to lymphedema generally improve over time. Sleeping with the upper body in an elevated position can use gravity to speed the process of lymph fluid drainage. A lymphedema treatment specialist can perform and teach manual lymph drainage that can help in reducing edema. Manual lymph drainage involves a special type of gentle skin massage to help blocked lymphatic fluid drain properly into the bloodstream. Movement and exercise are also important in aiding lymphatic drainage. A head and neck lymphedema therapist can teach the patient specific exercises to improve the range of head and neck motion.

A head and neck lymphedema therapist can select non-elastic bandages or compression garments that are worn at home. These place gentle pressure on the affected areas to help move the lymph fluid and prevent it from refilling and swelling. Application of bandages should be done as directed by a specialist. There are several options, depending on the location of the lymphedema to improve comfort and avoid complications from pressure on the neck.

There are also exercises that can reduce the neck tightness and increase the range of neck motion. One needs to perform these exercises throughout life to maintain good neck mobility. This is especially true if the stiffness is due to radiation. Receiving treatment by experienced physical therapies who can also break down the fibrosis is very helpful. The earlier the intervention the better.

A new treatment modality that reduces lymphedema, fibrosis and neck muscle stiffness using *external laser* is also available. This method uses a low energy laser beam administered by an experienced physical therapist. The laser beam penetrates into the tissues where it is absorbed by cells and changes their metabolic processes. The beam is generated by the LTU-904 Portable Laser Therapeutic Unit. (http://www.stepup-speakout.org/Laser%20Brochure.pdf). This treatment can reduce the lymphedema in the neck and face and increase the range of motion in the head. It is a painless method that is done by placing the laser instrument at several locations over the neck for about 10 second intervals.

There are physical therapy experts in most communities who specialize in reducing swelling and edema. Consult one's surgeon to find out if physical therapy is a good therapeutic option for lymphedema.

The National Lympedema Network has a web site (http://www. lymphnet.org/resourceGuide/findTreatment.htm) that contains a list of lymphedema treatment specialists in North America, Europe and Australia.

A facial and neck guide of self administered massage is available at: http://www.aurorahealthcare.org/FYWB_pdfs/x23169.pdf

Skin numbness after surgery

The cervical lymph nodes, or glands, are generally surgically removed when the cancer is excised. When the surgeons remove these glands, they also cut some of the sensory nerves that supply the lower facial and neck skin. This creates numbness in the areas supplied by the severed nerves. Some of the numb areas may regain sensation in the months following the surgery, but other areas may remain permanently numb.

Most individuals become accustomed to the numbness and are able to prevent damage to the skin from sharp objects, heat or frost. Men learn not to injure the affected area when shaving by using an electric shaver.

The numb skin should be protected from sun burn by applying sunscreen and/or by shielding it with a garment. Frostbite can be prevented by covering the area with a scarf.

CHAPTER 6:

Methods of speaking after laryngectomy

Although total laryngectomy removes the entire larynx (vocal cords/ voice box), most laryngectomees can acquire a new way of speaking. About 85-90% of laryngectomees learn to speak using one of the three main methods of speaking described below. About ten percent do not communicate by speaking but can use computer-based or other methods to communicate.

Individuals normally speak by exhaling air from their lungs to vibrate their vocal cords. These vibration sounds are modified in the mouth by the tongue, lips, and teeth to generate the sounds that create speech. Although the vocal cords that are the source of the vibrating sounds are removed during total laryngectomy, other forms of speech can be created by using a new pathway for air and a different airway part to vibrate. Another method is to generate vibration by an artificial source placed on the outside of the throat or mouth and then using the mouth parts to form speech.

The method(s) used to speak again depend on the type of surgery. Some people may be limited to a single method, while others may have several choices.

Each method has unique characteristics, advantages and disadvantages. The goal of attaining a new way to speak is to meet the communication needs of each laryngectomee.

Speech and language pathologists (SLPs) can assist and guide laryngectomees in the proper use of the methods and/or devices they use to obtain the most understandable speech. Speech improves considerably between six months and one year after total laryngectomy. Active voice rehabilitation is associated with attaining better functional speech.

The three main methods of speaking after laryngectomy are:

1. Tracheoesophageal speech

In tracheoesophageal speech pulmonary air is exhaled from the trachea into the esophagus through a small silicone voice prosthesis that connects the two, and the vibrations are generated by the lower pharynx (Figure 2).

The voice prosthesis is inserted into the puncture (called tracheoesophageal puncture or TEP) created by the surgeon in the back of the neck stoma. The puncture is made at the back of the trachea (the windpipe) and goes into the esophagus (food tube). The hole between the trachea and esophagus can be done at the same time as the laryngectomy surgery (a primary puncture), or after healing from the surgery has occurred (a secondary puncture). A small tube, called a voice prosthesis, is inserted in this hole and prevents the puncture from closing. It has a one-way valve at the end on the esophagus side which allows air to go into the esophagus but prevents swallowed liquids from coming through the prosthesis and reaching the trachea and lungs.

Speaking is possible by diverting the exhaled air through the prosthesis into the esophagus by temporarily occluding the stoma: This can be done by sealing it with a finger or by pressing on a special Heat and Moisture Exchanger (HME) filter that is worn over the stoma. (See **HME advantages,** page 65) An HME partially restores the lost nasal functions. Some people use a "hands free" HME (automatic speaking valve) that is activated by speaking (See **Using hands free HME,** page 69).

After occlusion of the stoma exhaled lung air moves through the prosthesis into the esophagus causing the walls and top of the esophagus to vibrate. These vibrations are used by the mouth (tongue, lips, teeth, etc.) to create the sounds of speech.

There are two different basic types of voice prosthesis: the patient-changed type, designed to be changed by the laryngectomee or by another person, and the indwelling type, designed to be changed by a medical professional (an otolaryngologist or SLP).

The HME or hands free valve can be attached in front of the tracheostoma in different ways: by means of an adhesive housing (or base plate) that is taped or glued to the skin in front of the stoma, or by means of a laryngectomy tube or stoma button that is placed inside the stoma.

Patients who use a voice prosthesis had the best results in speech intelligibility six months and one year after total laryngectomy.

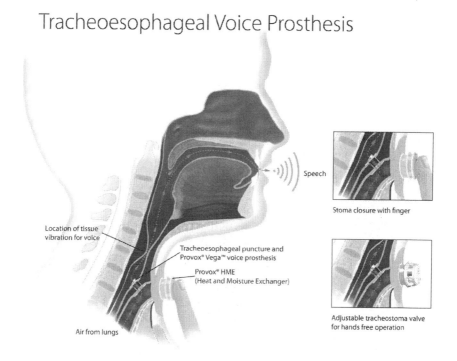

Tracheoesophageal Voice Prosthesis

Speech

Stoma closure with finger

Location of tissue vibration for voice

Tracheoesophageal puncture and Provox® Vega™ voice prosthesis

Provox® HME (Heat and Moisture Exchanger)

Adjustable tracheostoma valve for hands free operation

Air from lungs

Figure 2: Tracheoesophageal speech

2. Esophageal speech

In esophageal speech the vibrations are generated by air that is "belched" out from the esophagus (Figure 3). This method does not require any instrumentation.

Of the three major types of speech following laryngectomy, esophageal speech usually takes the longest to learn. However, it has several advantages, not the least of which includes the freedom from dependency on devices and instrumentation.

Some SLPs are familiar with esophageal speech and can assist laryngectomees in learning this method. Self-help books and tapes can also help in learning this method of speech.

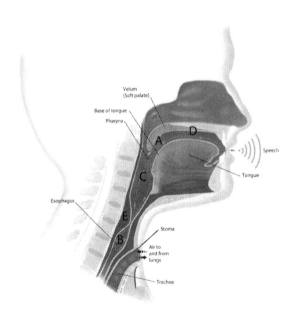

Figure 3: Esophageal speech

3. Electrolarynx or artificial larynx speech

The vibrations in this speech method are generated by an external battery operated vibrator (called an electrolarynx or artificial larynx) which is usually placed on the cheek or under the chin (Figure 4).

It makes a buzzing vibration that reaches the throat and mouth of the user. The person then modifies the sound using his/her mouth to generate the speech sounds.

There are two main methods to deliver the vibration sounds created by an artificial larynx into the throat and mouth (intra orally). One is directly into the mouth by a straw-like tube and the other through the skin of the neck or face. In the last method, the electrolarynx (EL) is held against the face or neck.

ELs are often used by laryngectomees shortly after their laryngectomy while they are still hospitalized. Because of the neck swelling and post surgical stitches the intra oral route of delivery of vibration is preferred at that time. Many laryngectomees can learn other methods of speaking later. However, they can still use an EL as a back-up in case they encounter problems with their other speaking methods.

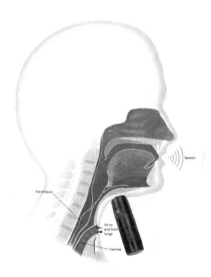

Figure 4: Electrolarynx or artificial larynx speech

Other methods of speech

A pneumatic artificial larynx (also called Tokyo Larynx) is also available to generate speech. This method uses lung air to vibrate a reed or rubber material that produces a sound (Picture 1). The device's cup is placed over the stoma and its tube is inserted into the mouth. The sound generated is injected into the mouth through the tube. It does not use any batteries and is relatively inexpensive.

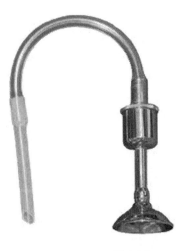

Picture 1: Pneumatic artificial larynx

Those who are unable to use any of the above methods can use computer generated speech using either a standard laptop computer or a single purpose speech aid. The user types what he/she wants to say onto a keyboard, and the computer speaks out loud what has been typed. Some cell phones can operate in the same manner.

Diaphragmatic breathing and speech

Diaphragmatic breathing (also called abdominal breathing) is the act of breathing slowly and deeply into one's lungs by using the diaphragm muscle rather than by using one's rib cage muscles. When breathing using the diaphragm, the abdomen, rather than the chest is expands. This method of breathing allows for greater utilization of the lung capacity to obtain oxygen and dispose of bicarbonate gasses. Neck breathers are often shallow breathers who use a relatively smaller portion of their lung capacity. Becoming accustomed to inhaling by using the diaphragm can increase one's stamina and also improve esophageal and tracheoesophageal speech.

Increasing the voice volume using a voice amplifier

One of the problems encountered when using trachoesophageal or esophageal speech is the weakness of the volume. Using a waistband voice amplifier can enable one to speak with less effort and can allow one to be heard even in noisy places. It can also prevent breakage of the stoma's housing seal because the laryngecomee who uses tracheoesophageal speech does not need to create a strong expiratory air pressure to exhale air though the voice prosthesis.

Speaking over the phone

Speaking over the phone is often difficult for laryngectomees. Their voice is sometimes hard to understand and some individuals may even hang up the phone when they hear them.

It is best to inform the other party about the speaking difficulties of the laryngectomee by first asking them "can you hear me?". This may enable the larynngectomee to inform and explain to their party about their speaking difficulties.

There are phones available that can amplify the outgoing voice, making it easier for the laryngectomee to be heard and understood.

A nationwide phone service allows a person whose speech may be difficult to understand to communicate over the telephone with the help of a specially trained Communications Assistant. No special telephone is needed for this calling option. The three digit number 711 can be used as a shortcut to access Telecommunications Relay Services (TRS) anywhere in the U.S. TRS facilitates telephone conversations by one or more people who have speech and hearing disabilities. All telecommunications carriers in the U.S., including wire-line, wireless and pay phone providers must provide 711 services.

Sending written messages through mobile phones (smart phones, or cell phones) can help laryngectommees communicate in noisy places or when they have other communication difficulties.

CHAPTER 7:

Mucus and respiratory care

Mucus production is the body's way of protecting and maintaining the health of the trachea (windpipe) and lungs. It serves to lubricate these airways and keep them moist. After a laryngectomy, the trachea opens at the stoma and laryngectomees are no longer able to cough up mucus into their mouth and then swallow it, or blow their nose. It is still very important to cough and clear one's mucus; however, this must be done through the stoma.

Coughing up mucus through the stoma is the only means by which laryngectomees can keep their trachea and lungs clear of dust, dirt, organisms, and other contaminants that get into the airway. Whenever an urge to cough or sneeze emerges laryngectomee must quickly remove their stoma cover or Heat and Moisture Exchanger (HME) and use a tissue or handkerchief to cover their stoma to catch the mucus.

The best mucus consistency is clear, or almost clear, and watery. Such consistency is, however, not easy to maintain because of changes in the environment and weather. Steps can be routinely taken to maintain a healthy mucus production as shown below.

Mucus production and increasing air humidity

Prior to becoming a laryngectomee, an individual's inhaled air is warmed to body temperature, humidified and cleansed of organisms and dust particles by the upper part of the respiratory system. Since these functions do not occur following laryngectomy, it is important to restore the lost functions previously provided by the upper part of the respiratory system.

Following laryngectomy the inhaled air does not get humidified by passing through the nose and mouth; accordingly, tracheal dryness, irritation and overproduction of mucus develop. Fortunately, the trachea becomes more tolerant to dry air over time. However, when the humidity level is too low the trachea can dry out, crack, and produce some bleeding. If the bleeding is significant or does not respond to increase in humidity, a physician should be consulted. And if the amount or color of the mucus is concerning, one should contact a physician.

Restoring the humidification of the inhaled air reduces the overproduction of mucus to an adequate level. This will decrease the chances for coughing unexpectedly and plugging the HME. Increasing the home humidity to 40-50% relative humidity (not higher) can help in decreasing mucus production and keeping the stoma and trachea from drying out, cracking and bleeding. In addition to being painful, these cracks can also become pathways for infections.

Steps to achieve better humidification include:

- Wearing an HME 24/7 which keeps the tracheal moisture higher and preserves the heat inside the lungs

- Wetting the soma cover to breathe moist air (in those who wear a stoma cover). Although less effective than an HME, dampening the foam filter or stoma cover with clean plain water can also assist in increasing humidification.

- Drinking enough fluid to keep well hydrated

- Inserting 3-5 cc saline into the trachea into stoma at least twice a day

- Taking a steamy shower or breathing in water vapor from a tea kettle (from a safe distance) can also reduce dryness

- Using a humidifier in the house to achieve about 40-50% humidity and getting a hygrometer to monitor the humidity. This is important both in the summer when air conditioning is used, and in the winter when heating is used

- Breathing steam generated by boiling water or a hot shower

There are two types of portable humidifiers - the steam and evaporative ones. A digital humidity gauge (called a hygrometer) can assist in controlling the humidity levels. Over time as the airway adjusts, the need to always use a humidifier may decrease.

Caring for the airway and neck especially in a cold winter and in high altitude

Winter and high altitude can be rough for laryngectomees. The air at high altitude is thinner and colder and therefore dryer. Before a laryngectomy, air is inhaled through the nose where is becomes warm and moist before entering the lungs. After a laryngectomy the air is no longer inhaled through the nose and enters the trachea directly through the stoma. Cold air is dryer than warm air and more irritating to the trachea. This is because cold air contains less humidity and therefore can dry the trachea and cause bleeding.

The mucus can also become dry and plug the trachea.

Breathing cold air can also have an irritating effect on the airway causing the smooth muscle that surrounds the airway to contract (bronchospasm). This decreases the size of the airway and makes it hard to get the air in and out of the lungs, thus increasing shortness of breath.

Care for the airway includes all the steps described in the previous section as well as:

- Coughing out or suctioning the mucus using a suction machine to clean the airway

- Avoiding exposure to cold, dry or dusty air

- Avoiding dust, irritants and allergens

- When exposed to cold air, consider covering the stoma with a jacket (by zipping it all the way) or a loose scarf and breathing into the space between the jacket and the body to warm the inhaled air.

- Preventing water from getting into the stoma when showering (see below)

Following a laryngectomy which involves neck dissection most individuals develop areas of numbness in their neck, chin and behind the ears. Consequently, they cannot sense cold air and can develop frostbite at these sites. It is therefore important to cover these areas with a scarf or warm garment.

Using suction machine for mucus plugs

A suction machine is often ordered for a laryngectomee prior to leaving the hospital for use at home. It can be used to suction out mucus when one is unable to cough it out and/or to remove a mucus plug. A mucus plug can develop when the mucus become thick and sticky, creating a plug that blocks part or, infrequently, even the whole airway.

The plug can cause a sudden and unexplained shortness of breath. A suction machine can be used in these circumstances to remove the plug. It should therefore be readily available to treat such an emergency. Mucus plugs may also be removed by using a saline "bullet" (0.9% sterile salt water in a plastic tube) or by squirting saline solution into the stoma. The saline can loosen the plug that can be coughed out. This condition may become a medical emergency and, if the plug is not successfully removed after several attempts, dialing 911 may be life saving.

Coughing blood

Blood in the mucus can originate from several sources. The most common is from a scratch just inside the stoma. The scratch can be caused by trauma while cleaning the stoma. The blood generally appears bright red. Another common cause of coughing blood in a laryngectomee is irritation of the trachea because of dryness which is common during the winter. It is advisable to maintain a home environment with adequate humidity levels (about 40-50%) to help minimize drying the trachea. Squirting sterile saline into the stoma can also help (See **Mucus production,** page 51).

Bloody sputum can also be a symptom of pneumonia, tuberculosis, lung cancer, or other lung problem.

Persistent coughing of blood should be evaluated by medical professionals. This may be urgent if it is associated with difficulties in breathing and/or pain.

Runny nose

Because laryngectomees and other neck breathers no longer breathe through their nose, their nasal secretions are not being dried by moving air. Consequently, the secretions drip out of the nose whenever large quantities of them are produced. This is especially common when one is exposed to cold and humid air or irritating smells. Avoiding these conditions can prevent a runny nose.

Wiping the secretion is the best practical solution. Laryngectomees using a voice prosthesis may be able to blow their nose by occluding the tracheostoma and divert air through the nose.

Respiratory rehabilitation

After a laryngectomy the inhaled air bypasses the upper part of the respiratory system and enters the trachea and lungs directly through the stoma. Laryngectomees therefore lose the part of the respiratory system that used to filter, warm and humidify the air they breathe.

The change in the way breathing is done also affects the efforts needed to breathe and potential lung functions. This requires adjustment and retraining. Breathing is actually easier for laryngectomees because there is less air flow resistance when the air bypasses the nose and mouth. Because it is easier to get air into the lungs, laryngectomees no longer need to inflate and deflate their lungs as completely as they did before. It is therefore not unusual for laryngectomees to develop reduced lung capacity and breathing capabilities.

There are several measures available to laryngectomees that can preserve and increase their lung capacity:

- The use of an HME can create resistance to air exchange. This forces the individual to fully inflate their lungs to get the needed amount of oxygen.

- Regular exercise under medical supervision and guidance. This can get the lungs to fully inflate and improve individuals' heart and breathing rates.

- Using diaphragmatic breathing. This method of breathing allows for greater utilization of the lung capacity. (See **Diaphragmatic breathing and speech,** page 48)

CHAPTER 8:

Stoma care

A stoma is an opening that connects a portion of the body cavity to the outside environment. A stoma is created after a laryngectomy to generate a new opening for the trachea in the neck, thus connecting the lungs to the outside. Caring for the stoma to insure its patency and health is crucial.

General care

It is very important to cover the stoma at all times in order to prevent dirt, dust, smoke, micro-organisms, etc., from getting into the trachea and lungs.

There are various kinds of stoma covers. The most effective ones are called Heat and Moisture Exchangers (HME) because they create a tight seal around the stoma. In addition to filtering dirt, HMEs preserve some of the moisture and heat inside the respiratory tract and prevent the person from losing them. The HME therefore assist in restoring the temperature, moisture and cleanliness of the inhaled air to the condition before the laryngectomy.

The stoma often shrinks during the first weeks or months after it is created. To prevent it from closing completely, a tracheostomy or laryngectomy tube is initially left in the stoma 24 hours a day. Over time this duration is gradually reduced. It is often left overnight until there is no more shrinking.

Stoma care when using a base plate or adhesive housing: The skin around the stoma can become irritated because of repeated gluing and removal of the housing. The materials used to remove the old housing and prepare for the new one can irritate the skin. Removal of the old housing can also irritate the skin especially when it is glued.

An adhesive removal wipe containing liquid (e.g., Remove™, Smith & Nephew, Inc. Largo Fl 33773) can assist in removing the base plate or housing. It is placed at the edge of the housing and helps the housing detach from the skin when it is lifted off. Wiping the area with Remove ™ cleans the site from remnants of the seal used to glue the housing. It is important to wipe off the leftover Remove ™ with an alcohol wipe so that it will not irritate the skin. When a new housing is used wiping off the Remove ™ prevents it from interfering with placing glue again.

It is generally not recommended to leave the housing on for more than 48 hours. Some individuals, however, keep the housing much longer, and replace it when it becomes loose or dirty. In some people the removal of the adhesive is more irritating than the adhesives. In the event the skin is irritated, it is better to leave the housing on only for 24 hours. If the skin is irritated, it may be advisable to give the skin a rest for a day or until the area heals and cover the stoma only with a rigid base without any glue or with a foam cover. There are special hydrocolloid adhesives that allow use on sensitive skin.

It is important to use a liquid film-forming skin protecting dressing (i.e., Skin Prep ™, Smith & Nephew, Inc. Largo Fl 33773) before placing the glue.

Stoma care when using tracheostomy tube: The buildup of mucus and the rubbing of the tracheostomy tube can irritate the skin around the stoma. The skin around the stoma should be cleaned at least twice a day to prevent odor, irritation and infection. If the area appears red, tender or smells bad, stoma cleaning should be performed more frequently. Contacting one's physician is advisable if a rash, unusual odor, and/or yellowish-green drainage appear around the stoma.

Skin irritation around the stoma

If the skin around the stoma becomes irritated and red, it is best to leave it uncovered and not expose it to any solvents for 1-2 days so that it can heal. Sometimes individuals can develop an irritation to some of the solvents used to prepare and glue an HME base plate (housing). Avoiding these solvents and finding others that do not cause irritation is helpful. Using a hydrocolloid adhesive is often a good solution for patients with sensitive skin.

If signs of infection such as open ulcers and redness are evident topical antibiotics can be useful. Seeking advice from one's physician is helpful especially if the lesion does not heal. The physician can obtain a bacterial culture of the affected area that can guide the choice of antimicrobial therapy.

Protecting the stoma from water when showering

It is important to prevent water from entering the stoma when taking a shower. A small amount of water in the trachea generally does not cause any harm and can be rapidly coughed out. However, inhalation of a large amount of water can be dangerous.

Methods to prevent water from entering the stoma are:

- Covering the stoma with the palm and not inhaling air when water is directed at the vicinity of the stoma.

- Wearing a bib with the plastic side out.

- Using a commercial device that covers the stoma.

- Wearing one's stoma cover, the base plate, or HME housing while showering may be sufficient especially if water flow is directed away from the stoma. Pausing air inhalation for a few seconds while washing the area close to the stoma is also helpful. Taking a shower at the end of the day just before removing the HME and its housing is a way to use the housing for water protection. This simple method can make taking a shower easier.

- When washing the hair, lowering the chin below the stoma by bending over.

Water and pneumonia

Laryngectomees are at risk of inhaling (aspirating) water that may not be free of bacteria. Tap water contains bacteria; the number of bacteria varies depending on the cleaning efficacy of the water treatment facilities and their source (e.g., well, lake, river, etc.). Pool water contains chloride that reduces, but never sterilizes the water. Sea water contains numerous bacteria; their nature and concentrations varies.

When unclean water gets into the lungs it can sometimes cause pneumonia. Developing aspiration pneumonia depends on how much water is inhaled and how much is coughed out, as well as on the individuals' immune system.

Preventing aspiration into the stoma

One of the major causes of respiratory emergency in a neck breather is the aspiration of thin paper tissue or paper towels into the trachea. This can be very dangerous and can cause asphyxiation. It usually happens after covering the stoma with a paper towel when coughing out sputum. Following the cough there is a very deep inspiration of air that can suck the paper back into the trachea. The way to prevent this is to use a cloth towel or a strong paper towel that does not break easily, even when moist. Thin tissues should be avoided.

Another way to prevent aspiration of paper tissues is to hold one's breath until one has completely finished wiping off the sputum and removed the paper tissue or paper towel from the stoma area.

Aspiration of other foreign material should also be prevented by covering the stoma at all times by an HME, foam cover, or stoma cover.

Aspiration of water into the stoma while taking a shower can be prevented by wearing a device that covers the stoma (see above). One can keep the HME on while showering and/or avoid breathing in when water is directed at the stoma's site.

Taking a bath in a tub can be done safely as long as the water level does not reach the stoma. The areas above the stoma should be washed with a soapy washcloth. It is important to prevent soapy water from entering the stoma.

CHAPTER 9:

Heat moisture exchanger (HME) care

Heat and moisture exchanger (HME) serve as stoma covers and create a tight seal around the stoma. In addition to filtering dust and other large airborne particles, HMEs preserve some of the moisture and heat inside the respiratory tract and prevent their loss, and adds resistance to the airflow. HME assist in restoring the temperature, moisture and cleanliness of the inhaled air to the same condition as before laryngectomy.

HME advantages

It is very important that laryngectoees wear an HME. In the United States, the HMEs are available through Atos Medical and InHealth Technologies (Picture 2). The HME can be attached by using an intraluminal device inserted into the trachea or stoma, that includes laryngectomy or tracheostomy tubes, Barton Mayo Button™ and/or Lary Button™. The can also be inserted into a housing or a base plate attached to the skin around the stoma.

HME cassettes are designed to be removed and replaced on a daily basis. The foam media in the cassettes are treated with agents that have antimicrobial properties and help to retain moisture in the lungs. They should not be washed and reused because these agents lose their effectiveness over time or when rinsed by water or other cleaning agents.

The HME captures the warm, moistened, and humidified air upon exhalation. It can be impregnated with chlorhexidine (anti-bacterial agent), sodium chloride (NaCl), calcium chloride salts (traps moisture), activated charcoal (absorbs volatile fumes), and is disposable after 24 hours of use.

The HME advantages also include: increasing the moisture within the lungs (subsequently leading to less mucus production), decreasing the viscosity of the airway secretions, decreasing risk of mucus plugs, and re-instating the normal airway resistance to the inhaled air which preserves the lung capacity.

In addition, a special HME-combined with an electrostatic filter also reduces the inhalation (and exhalation/transfer) of bacteria, viruses, dust and pollen. Inhaling less pollen can reduce the airway irritation during high allergens season. Wearing an HME with filter may reduce the risk of getting or transferring viral and bacterial infection, especially in crowded or closed places. A new HME filter designed to filter potential respiratory pathogens is available (Provox Micron ™, Atos Medical).

It is important to realize that simple stoma covers, such as a laryngofoam™ filter, ascot, bandana, etc., do not provide the same benefits to a laryngectomee as an HME filter.

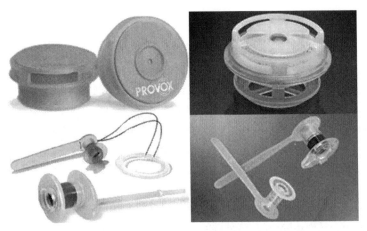

Picture 2: Voice prosthesis (below) and HMEs (above) produced by Atos Medical (Provox) and InHealth

The effect of an HME on breathing as a laryngectomee

Laryngectomy compromises the respiratory system by allowing the inhaled air to bypass the nose and upper airways which normally provide humidification, filtration and warmth. It also reduces the resistance and the effort needed for inhalation by removing air resistance and shortening the distance the air travels to the lung. This means that laryngectomees do not have to work as hard to get air past the upper part of the system (nose, nasal passages, and throat), and their lungs do not have to inflate as much as they did before unless the person works to retain their capacity through exercise and other methods. An HME increases the resistance to inhaled air and therefore increases inhalation efforts, thus preserving previous lung capacity.

Placing an HME base plate (housing)

The key to prolonging the use of am HME's base plate (housing) is not only properly gluing it in place, but also removing the old adhesives and glue from the skin, cleaning the area around the stoma and applying new layers of adhesive and glue. Careful preparation of the skin is very important (Picture 3).

In some individuals the shape of the neck around the stoma makes it difficult to fit a housing or a base plate. There are several types of housing; a speech and language pathologist (SLP) can assist in selecting the best one. Finding the best HME housing may take trial and error. Over time, as the post surgical swelling subsides and the area around the stoma reshapes itself, the type and size of the housing may change.

Below are the suggested instructions on how to place the housing for the HME. Throughout the process it is important to wait patiently and allow the liquid film-forming skin protecting dressing (i.e., Skin Prep™ Smith & Nephew, Inc. Largo, Fl 33773) and silicone skin adhesive to dry before applying the next item or placing the housing. This takes time, but it is important to follow these instructions:

1. Clean the old glue with an adhesive removal wipe (e.g., Remove™, Smith & Nephew, Inc. Largo, Fl 33773).

2. Wipe off the Remove™ with an alcohol wipe. (if you do not do this, the Remove™ will interfere with the new adhesive).

3. Wipe the skin with a wet towel.

4. Wipe the skin with the wet towel with soap.

5. Wash away the soap with a wet towel and thoroughly dry.

6. Apply Skin Prep™ and let it dry for 2-3 minutes.

7. For extra adhesion apply silicone skin adhesive or Skin-Tac ™ wipe (Torbot, Cranston, Rhode Island, 20910) and let it dry for 3-4 minutes. (This is especially important for users of automatic speaking valve)

8. Attach the base plate (housing) for the HME at the best location to allow air flow and good attachment.

9. When using hands free HME wait for 5-30 minutes before speaking to allow the adhesive to "set".

Some SLPs recommend warming the housing prior to placement by rubbing it in the hands, holding it under the armpit for a few minutes, or by blowing warm air on it with a hair drier. Be careful that the adhesive does not become too hot. Warming the adhesive is especially important when you use a hydrocolloid adhesive since the warmth activates the glue.

A video made by Steve Staton demonstrates the placement of the housing at http://www.youtube.com/watch?v=5Wo1z5_n1j8

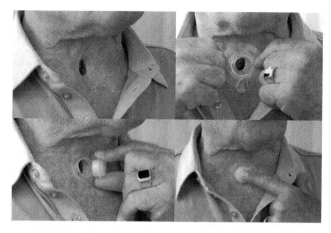

Picture 3: Placement of HME and its housing on a stoma

Using hands free HME

The hands free HME allows speaking without the need to manually press on the HME to close it off, thus blocking exhalation through the stoma and directing air to the voice prosthesis. This device frees one's hand and eases vocational and recreational possibilities. Note that when using a hands free HME more pressure is generated when air is exhaled thus potentially leading to a break in the HME housing's seal. Reducing the exhalation pressure when speaking, speaking slower and softly (almost whispering), and taking a breath after 5-7 words can prevent a break in the seal. Supporting it with a finger before needing to speak loud can also help. It is also important to quickly remove the device before coughing.

The air filter (also called cassette in Provox FreeHands HME) in the hands free device has to be changed on a regular basis (every 24 hours or sooner if it becomes dirty or covered with mucus). However, the HME device can be used for a long period of time (six months to a year) with proper use and cleaning. The hands free device requires initial adjustments to fit the laryngectomee's breathing and speaking abilities. Detailed instructions on how to use and care for the devices are provided by their manufacturers.

The key to speaking with a hands free HME is to learn how to speak without breaking the seal. Using diaphragmatic breathing allows for more air to be exhaled, thus reducing speaking efforts and increasing the number of words that can be articulated with each breath. This method prevents buildup of air pressure in the trachea which can break the housing's seal. It may take time and patience to learn how to speak in such a way, and guidance by a skilled SLP can be helpful.

It is very important to place the HME housing according to the steps outlined in the section on HME care (See **Placing an HME Housing,** page 67) including cleaning the area around the stoma with Remove™, alcohol, water and soap, placing Skin Prep™ and finally glue (Skin Tag™). Following these instructions can prolong the life of the housing and reduce the likelihood of an air leak through the seal.

Air inhalation is slightly more difficult when using a free hands HME as compared to a regular HME. It is possible to allow for greater amounts of air intake by rotating the valve counter-clockwise in both Atos FreeHands™ and InHealth HandsFree™ devices.

Despite the challenge of keeping the seal, many laryngectomees value the ability to speak in a more natural way and the freedom of using both hands. Some learn that it is possible to keep the seal much longer when they use a voice amplifier thus requiring less effort and generating less air pressure. (See **Increasing the voice using a voice amplifier,** page 49)

Wearing the HME overnight

Some HMEs are approved for wear 24/7 (i.e., Atos Medical). If the seal lasts, one can keep it overnight. If it does not last, it is possible to use an improvised base plate for the night period. An Atos Xtra BasePlate™ can be trimmed down by removing the outer soft part and leaving the inner rigid part. The plate is "sticky" and thus can cover the stoma without glue, even enabling one to speak. It is also possible to use the HME inserted in a LaryTube overnight.

Covering (hiding) the HME

Following laryngectomy, individuals breathe through a tracheostomy site that opens through a stoma on their neck. Most place an HME or a foam filter over the stoma to filter the inhaled air and maintain warmth and humidity in the upper airway. The covered stoma site is prominent and laryngectomees face a choice whether to cover the HME or filter with a garment, an ascot, or jewelry or to leave it uncovered.

The pros and cones of each choice:

Breathing may be easier without an additional cover which can interfere with air flow. Leaving the area exposed allows for easier access to the stoma for purpose of cleaning and maintenance and enables a rapid removal of the HME in case one needs to cough or sneeze. The urge to cough or sneeze is often very sudden and if the HME is not taken out quickly it can become clogged with mucus.

Exposing the site provides an unspoken explanation for the weak and rusty voice of many laryngectomees and encourages others to listen to them more attentively. It also makes it easier for health care providers to recognize the laryngectomee's unique anatomy in case emergency respiratory ventilation is needed. If this condition is not rapidly recognized ventilation may be administered through the mouth or nose rather than through the stoma. (See **Ensuring adequate urgent care of neck breathers including laryngectomees,** page 147)

Openly displaying the covered stoma site also reveals the person's medical history and the fact that he/she are cancer survivors who go on with their lives despite their handicap, cancer being the leading indication for a laryngectomy. Although there are many cancer survivors in the community, their identity is hidden from outward appearances.

Those who cover their stoma site with a stoma cover or cloth often do it because they do not want others to be distracted or offended by the site. They also do not want to expose anything that is disfiguring and want to be inconspicuous and appear as normal as possible. Covering the site is often more common among females who may be more concerned with their physical appearance. Some individuals feel that being a laryngectomee is only a small part of who they are as a person; they do not want to "advertise" it.

There are advantages and repercussions to each approach and the final selection is up to the individual.

CHAPTER 10:

Tracheoesophageal voice prosthesis use and care

A voice prosthesis is inserted through a previously created tracheoesophageal puncture (TEP) connecting the trachea and esophagus in those wishing to speak through tracheoesophageal speech. It enables the individual to exhale pulmonary air from the trachea into the esophagus through a silicone prosthesis that connects the two; the vibrations are generated by the lower pharynx.

Types of voice prosthesis

There are two types of voice prosthesis: an indwelling one that is installed and changed by a speech and language pathologist (SLP) or otolaryngologist and a patient-changed one.

The indwelling prosthesis generally lasts a longer time than the patient managed device. However, prosthesis eventually leak mostly because yeast and other microorganisms grow into the silicone leading to incomplete closure of the valve flap. When the valve flap does not close tight anymore, fluids can pass through the voice prosthesis (see below in **Causes of voice prosthesis leak section,** page 75).

An indwelling prosthesis can function well for weeks to months. However, some SLPs believe that it should be changed even when it does not leak after six months because, if left for a longer time, it can lead to dilatation of the puncture.

The patient managed voice prosthesis allows a greater degree of independence. It can be changed by the laryngectomee on a regular basis, (every one to two weeks). Some individuals change the prosthesis only after it starts leaking. The old prosthesis can be cleaned and reused several times.

A number of factors determine an individual's ability to use a patient managed prosthesis:

- The location of the puncture should be easily accessible; the site of the puncture may, however, migrate over time, making it less accessible.

- The laryngectomee should have adequate eyesight and good dexterity, enabling him/her to perform the procedure, and capable of following all the steps involved.

An indwelling voice prosthesis does not need to be replaced as frequently as a patient managed one.

Two videos made by Steve Staton explain how to change a patient-changed prosthesis:

http://www.youtube.com/watch?v=nF7cs4Q29WA&feature=channel_page

http://www.youtube.com/watch?v=UkeOQf_ZpUg&feature=relmfu

The main difference between the clinician-changed and patient-changed voice prosthesis is the size of the flanges. The larger size flanges on the clinician-changed devices make it harder to accidentally dislodge it. Another difference is that the insertion strap should not be removed from the patient-changeable prosthesis because it helps to anchor the prosthesis. There is generally no difference in voice quality between a clinician-changed and a patient-changed device.

What to do if the prosthesis leaks or is dislodged

If the prosthesis leaks or has become dislodged or has been removed accidentally, a patient-changed prosthesis can be inserted by those who carry an extra device. Alternatively, a red rubber catheter can be inserted into the TEP which can close within a few hours, to prevent closure. Inserting a catheter or a new prosthesis can prevent the need for a new TEP. Leakage of the prosthesis from the center (lumen) can be temporarily handled by inserting a plug (specific to the type and width of the prosthesis) until it can be changed.

It is advisable that individuals using a voice prosthesis carry a prosthesis plug and a catheter.

Causes of voice prosthesis leak

There are two patterns of voice prosthesis leak - leak through the prosthesis and leak around it.

Leakage **through the voice prosthesis** is predominantly due to situations in which the valve can no longer close tightly. This may be due the following: colonization of the valve by fungus; the flap valve may get stuck in the open position; a piece of food, mucus or hair (in those with a fee flap) stuck on the valve; or the device coming in contact with the posterior esophageal wall. Inevitably, all prostheses will fail by leaking through, whether from Candida colonization or simple mechanical failure.

If there is continuing leakage through the prosthesis from the time it is inserted, the problem is generally due to the fact that the flap valve remains open because of negative pressure generated by swallowing. This can be corrected by using a prosthesis that has a greater resistance. The trade-off is that having such a voice prosthesis may require more effort when speaking. It is, nevertheless, important to prevent chronic leakage into the lungs.

Leakage **around the voice prosthesis** is less common and is mainly due to trachea-esophageal puncture tract dilation or inability to grip the prosthesis. It has been linked to shorter prosthesis life time. It may occur when the puncture that houses the prosthesis widens. During insertion of the voice prosthesis, some dilation of the puncture takes place, but if the tissue is healthy and elastic, it should shrink back after a short time. The inability to contract may be associated with gastroesophageal reflux, poor nutrition, alcoholism, hypothyroidism, improper puncture placement, local granulation tissue, incorrectly fitted prosthesis, TEP tract trauma, recurrent or persistent local or distant cancer and radiation necrosis.

Leakage around the prosthesis can also occur if the prosthesis is too long for the user's tract. Whenever this occurs, the voice prosthesis moves back and forth in the tract (pistoning), thereby dilating the tract. The tract should be measured and a prosthesis of more appropriate length should be inserted. In this circumstance, leakage should resolve within 48 hours. If the tissue around the prosthesis does not heal around the shaft within this time period, comprehensive medical evaluation is warranted to determine the cause of the problem.

Another cause of leakage around the prosthesis is the presence of narrowing (stricture) of the esophagus. The narrowing of the esophagus forces the laryngectomee to swallow harder using greater force, so that the food/liquid goes through the stricture. The excess swallowing pressure pushes the food/liquid around the prosthesis.

Several procedures have been used to treat persistent leakage around the prosthesis. These include temporary removal of the prosthesis and replacement with a smaller-diameter catheter to encourage spontaneous shrinkage; a purse-string suture around the puncture; injection of gel, collagen or micronized AlloDerm® (LifeCell, Branchburg, N.J. 08876); cautery with silver nitrate or electocautery; autologous fat transplantation; and inserting a larger prosthesis to stop the leak. Treatment of reflux (the most common cause of leakage) can allow the esophageal tissue to heal.

Increasing the diameter of the prosthesis is generally not recommended.

Generally a larger diameter voice prosthesis is heavier than a smaller one, and the weakened tissue is often not able to support a bigger device, making the problem even worse. However, some believe that using a larger diameter prosthesis reduces the speaking pressure (larger diameter allows better airflow) which allows greater tissue healing to occur while the underlying cause (most often reflux) is treated.

The use of prosthesis with a larger esophageal and/or tracheal flange may be helpful, as the flange acts as a washer to seal the prosthesis against the walls of the esophagus and/or trachea, thus preventing leakage.

Both types of leakage can cause excessive, strenuous, coughing which may lead to the development of abdominal wall and inguinal hernias. The leaked fluid can enter the lungs and causing aspiration pneumonia. Any leakage can be confirmed by direct visualization of the prosthesis while drinking colored liquid. If leakage occurs and cannot be corrected after brushing and flushing the voice prosthesis, it should be changed as soon as possible.

With the passage of time, a voice prosthesis generally tends to last longer before it begins to leak. This is because the swelling and increased mucus production are reduced as the airway adapts to the new condition. Improvement is also due to better prosthesis management by laryngectomees as they familiarize themselves with their device.

Patients with a TEP need to be followed by a SLP because of normal changes in the tracheo-esophageal tract. Re-sizing of the tract may be needed as it can change in length and diameter with time. The length and diameter of the prosthesis puncture generally change over time as the swelling generated by creation of the fistula, surgery, and radiation gradually decreases. This requires repeated measurements of the length and diameter of the puncture tract by the SLP who can select a properly sized prosthesis.

One of the advantages of having a voice prosthesis is that it can assist in dislodging food stuck in a narrow throat. When food get stuck above the prosthesis, trying to speak or blowing air through the voice prosthesis can sometimes force the stuck food upward and relieve the obstruction. (See **How to remove or swallow food that is stuck in the throat or esophagus,** page 87)

The prosthesis may have to be changed if there is an alteration in the quality of the voice, especially when the voice becomes weaker or one needs more respiratory effort to speak. This may be due to yeast growth which interferes with the opening of the valve.

Preventing the voice prosthesis from leaking

It is advisable to clean the voice prosthesis' inner lumen at least twice a day and after each meal.

Proper cleaning may prevent and/or stop leakage through the voice prosthesis:

1. Before using the brush provided by the manufacturer, dip it in a cup of hot water and leave it there for a few seconds.

2. Insert the brush into the prosthesis (not too deep) and twist it around a few times to clean the inside of the device.

3. Take the brush out and rinse it with hot water and repeat the process 2-3 times until no material is brought out by the brush. Because the brush is dipped in hot water one should be careful not to insert it beyond the voice prosthesis inner valve to avoid traumatizing the esophagus with excessive heat.

4. Flush the voice prosthesis twice using the bulb provided by the manufacturer using warm (not hot!) potable water. To avoid damage to the esophagus sip the water first to make sure that the water temperature is not too high.

Warm water works better than room temperature water in cleansing the prosthesis probably because it dissolves the dry secretions and mucus and perhaps even flushes away (or even kills) some of the yeast colonies that had formed on the prosthesis.

What to do if the indwelling voice prosthesis leaks

A leak can take place when a piece of dry mucus, a food particle, or hair (in those with a free flap) prevents a complete closure of the prosthesis's valve. Cleaning the prosthesis by brushing and flushing it with warm water (see the previous section) can remove these obstructions and stop the leakage.

If the leakage through the voice prosthesis happens within three days after its insertion it may be due to a defective prosthesis or one that was not placed correctly. It takes some time for the yeast to grow. If the prosthesis leaks when new, it is due to another cause. In addition to brushing and flushing with warm water, cautiously rotating the prosthesis a couple of times to dislodge any debris may help. If the leak persists the voice prosthesis should be replaced.

The easiest way of temporarily stopping the leak until the voice prosthesis can be changed is to use a plug. A plug is specific for the type and width of each voice prosthesis. It is a good idea to obtain a plug from the prosthesis' manufacturer and have it handy. Sealing the prosthesis will prevent speaking, but it allows eating and drinking without leakage. The plug can be removed after eating and drinking and reinserted as needed. This is a temporary solution until the voice prosthesis is replaced.

It is important to stay well hydrated despite the leakage. Avoiding fluid losses in hot weather through perspiration by staying in an air-conditioned environment and ingesting liquids in a way that is less likely to leak are helpful. Drinks that contain caffeine increase urination and should be avoided. Viscous fluids tend not to leak and consuming them can provide essential liquids despite the leak. Many food items that contain large amount of liquids are more viscous (e.g., jelly, soup, oat meal, toast dipped in milk, yogurt) and are therefore less likely to leak through the prosthesis. On the other hand coffee and carbonated drinks are more likely to leak. Fruits and vegetables contain large amount of water (e.g., watermelon, apples, etc). The way to find out what works is to cautiously try any of these.

Another method to reduce the leak until the prosthesis can be changed that may work for some individuals is to try and swallow the liquid as if it is a food item. Such maneuver is less likely to lead to fluid leakage through the voice prosthesis.

These measures can be used to keep well-hydrated and nourished until the voice prosthesis can be changed.

Cleaning the voice prosthesis

It is recommended that the voice prosthesis be cleaned at least twice a day, (morning and evening), and preferably after eating (see: **Preventing** the: **Voice prosthesis from leaking,** page 78) because this is the time when food and mucus can become trapped there. Cleaning is especially helpful after eating sticky food or whenever one's voice is weak.

Initially, the mucus around the prosthesis should be cleaned using tweezers, preferably with rounded tips. Following that the manufacturer-provided brush should be inserted into the prosthesis and twisted back and forth. The brush should be thoroughly washed with warm water after each cleaning. The prosthesis is then flushed twice with warm (not hot) water using the manufacturer's provided bulb.

The flushing bulb should be introduced into the prosthesis opening while applying slight pressure to completely seal off the opening. The angle that one should place the tip of the bulb varies between individuals. (The SLP can provide instructions how to choose the best angle.) Flushing the prosthesis should be done gently because using too much pressure can lead to splashing of water into the trachea. If flushing with water is problematic, the flush can also be used with air.

The manufacturers of each voice prosthesis brush and flushing bulb provide directions on how to clean them and when they should be discarded. The brush should be replaced when its threads become bent or worn out.

The prosthesis brush and flushing bulb should be cleaned with hot water, when possible and soap and dried with a towel after every use. One way to keep them clean is to place them on a clean towel and expose them to sunlight for a few hours, on a daily basis. This takes advantage of the antibacterial power of the sun's ultraviolet light to reduce the number of bacteria and fungi.

Placing 2-3 cc of sterile saline in the trachea at least twice a day (and more if the air is dry), wearing an HME 24/7 and using a humidifier can keep the mucus moist and reduce the clogging of the voice prosthesis.

Preventing yeast growth in the voice prosthesis

Overgrowth of yeast is one cause of a voice prosthesis leaking and thus failing. Nevertheless, it takes some time for yeast to grow in a newly installed voice prosthesis and form colonies that prevent its valve's from closing completely. Accordingly, failures immediately after voice prosthesis installation are unlikely due to yeast growth.

The presence of yeast should be established by the person who changes the failing voice prosthesis. This can be done by observing the typical yeast (Candida) colonies that prevent the valve from closing and, if possible, by sending a specimen from the voice prosthesis for fungal culture.

Mycostatin (an antifungal agent) is often used to prevent voice prosthesis failure due to yeast. It is available with a prescription in the form of a suspension or tablets. The tablets can be crushed and dissolved in water.

Automatically administering anti-fungal therapy just because one assumes that yeast is the cause of voice prosthesis failure may be inappropriate. It is expensive, may lead to the yeast developing resistance to the agent, and may cause unnecessary side effects.

There are, however, exceptions to this rule. These include the administration of preventive anti-fungal agents to diabetics; those receiving antibiotics; chemotherapy or steroids; and those where colonization with yeast is evident (coated tongue etc.).

There are several methods that help prevent yeast from growing on the voice prosthesis:

- Reduce the consumption of sugars in food and drinks. If you consume them, brush your teeth well after consuming sugary foods and/or drinks.

- Brush your teeth well after every meal and especially before going to sleep.

- Diabetics should maintain adequate blood sugar levels.

- Take antibiotics only if they are needed.

- After using an oral suspension of an antifungal agent, wait for 30 minutes to let it work and then brush your teeth. This is because some of these suspensions contain sugar.

- Dip the voice prosthesis brush in a small amount of mycostatin suspension and brush the inner voice prosthesis before going to sleep. (A homemade suspension can be made by dissolving a quarter of a mycostatin tablet in 3-5 cc water). This would leave some of the suspension inside the voice prosthesis. The unused suspension should be discarded. Do not to place too much mycostatin in the prosthesis to prevent dripping into the trachea. Speaking a few words after placing the suspension will push it towards the inner part of the voice prosthesis.

- Consume probiotics by eating active-culture yogurt and/or a probiotic preparation

- Gently brush the tongue if it is coated with yeast (white plaques)

- Replace the toothbrush after overcoming a yeast problem to prevent re colonizing with yeasts

- Keep the prosthesis brush clean

The use of *Lactobacillus acidophilus* to prevent yeast overgrowth

A probiotic that is often used to prevent yeast overgrowth is a preparation containing the viable bacteria *Lactobacillus acidophilus*. There is no FDA approved indication to use *L. acidophilus* to prevent yeast growth. This means that there were no controlled studies to ensure its safety and efficacy. *L. acidophilus* preparations are sold as a nutritional supplement and not as a medication. The recommended dosage of *L. acidophilus* is between 1 and 10 billion bacteria. Typically, *L. acidophilus* tablets contain somewhere within this recommended amount of bacteria. Dosage suggestions vary by tablet, but generally it is advised to take between one and three *L. acidophilus* tablets daily.

Although generally believed to be safe with few side effects, oral preparations of *L. acidophilus* should be avoided in people with intestinal damage, a weakened immune system, or with overgrowth of intestinal bacteria. In these individuals this bacterium can cause serious and sometimes life threatening complications. This is why individuals should consult their physician whenever this live bacteria is ingested. It is especially important in those with the above conditions.

CHAPTER 11:

Eating, swallowing, and smelling

Eating, swallowing, and smelling are not the same after laryngectomy. This is because radiation and surgery create permanent lifelong changes. Radiation therapy can cause fibrosis of the muscles of mastication which can lead to the inability to open one's mouth (trismus or lockjaw) making eating more difficult. Eating and swallowing difficulties can also be generated by a decrease in saliva production and a narrowing of the esophagus, plus a lack of peristalsis in those with flap reconstruction. Smelling is also affected because inhaled air bypasses the nose.

This chapter describes the manifestations and treatment of the eating and smelling challenges faced by laryngectomees. These include swallowing problem, food reflux, esophageal strictures, and smelling difficulties.

Maintaining adequate nutrition as a laryngectomee

Eating may be a lifelong challenge for laryngectomees. This is because of swallowing difficulties, decreased production of saliva (which lubricates food and eases mastication), and an alteration in one's ability to smell.

The need to consume large quantities of fluid while eating can make it difficult to ingest large meals. This is because when liquids fill the stomach there is less room left for food. Because liquids are absorbed within a relatively short period of time, laryngectomees end up having multiple small meals rather than fewer large ones. The consumption of large quantities of liquid makes them urinate very frequently throughout the day and night. This can interfere with one's sleep pattern and can cause tiredness and irritability. Those who suffer from heart problems (e.g., congestive heart failure) may experience problems due to overloading their bodies with excess fluid.

Consuming food that stays longer in the stomach (e.g., proteins such as white cheese, meat, nuts) can reduce the number of daily meals, thus reducing the need to drink liquids.

It is important to learn how to eat without ingesting excessive amounts of liquids. For example, relieving swallowing difficulties can reduce the need to consume fluids, while consuming fewer liquids prior to bedtime can improve sleeping pattern.

Nutrition can be improved by:

- Ingesting adequate, but not too much liquid

- Drinking less liquid in the evening

- Consuming "healthy" food

- Consuming a low carbohydrate and high protein diet (high sugar enhances yeast colonization)

- Requesting dietitian assistance

It is essential to make sure a laryngectomee follows an adequate and balanced nutrition plan that contains the correct ingredients, despite difficulties with their eating. A low carbohydrate and high protein diet that includes vitamins and minerals supplements is important. The assistance of nutritionists, speech and language pathologists (SLPs), and physicians in ensuring that one maintains adequate weight is very helpful.

How to remove (or swallow) food that is stuck in the throat or esophagus

Some laryngectomees experience recurrent episodes of food becoming stuck in the back of their throat or esophagus and prevents them from swallowing.

Clearing the stuck food can be accomplished using these methods:

1. First do not panic. Remember that you cannot suffocate because, as a laryngectomee, your esophagus is completely separate from your trachea.

2. Try to drink some liquid (preferably warm) and attempt to force the food down by increasing the pressure in your mouth. If this does not work -

3. If you speak through a tracheoesophageal puncture (TEP), try to speak. This way the air you blow through the voice prosthesis may push the food above the TEP into the back of your throat, relieving the obstruction. Try this first standing up and if it does not work bend over a sink and try to speak. If this does not work –

4. Bend forward (over a sink or hold a tissue or cup over the mouth), lowering your mouth below the chest and applying pressure over your abdomen with your hand. This forces the contents of the stomach upward and may clear the obstruction.

These methods work for most people. However, everyone is different and one needs to experiment and find the methods that best work for them. Swallowing does, however, get better in many laryngectomees over time.

Some laryngectomees report success in removing the obstruction by gently massaging their throat, walking for a few minutes, jumping up on their feet, sitting and standing several times, hitting their chest or the back, using a suction machine with the catheter paced in the back of their throat, or just waiting for a while until the food is able to descend into the stomach by itself.

If nothing works and the food is still stuck in the back of the throat it may be necessary to be seen by an otolaryngologist or go to an emergency room to have the obstruction removed.

Food and stomach acid reflux

Most laryngectomees are prone or develop gastroesophageal reflux disease, or GERD.

There are two muscular bands or sphincters in the esophagus that prevent reflux. One band is located where the esophagus enters the stomach and the other is behind the larynx at the beginning of the esophagus in the neck. The lower esophageal sphincter often becomes compromised when there is a hiatus hernia which in more than three quarters people over seventy. During a laryngectomy, the sphincter in the upper esophageal sphincter (the cricopharyngeus) which normally prevents food from returning to the mouth is removed. This leaves the upper part of the esophagus flaccid and always open which may result in the reflux of stomach contents up into the throat and mouth. Therefore, regurgitation of stomach acid and food, especially in the first hour or so after eating, can occur when bending forward or lying down. This can also occur after forceful exhalation of air when those who use a TEP try to speak.

Taking medications that reduce stomach acidity such as antacids and proton pump inhibitors (PPI), can alleviate some of the side effects of reflux, such as throat irritation, damage to the gums and bad taste. Not lying down after eating or drinking also helps prevent reflux. Eating small amounts of food multiple times causes less food reflux than eating large meals.

Symptoms and treatment of stomach acid reflux. Acid reflux occurs when the acid that is normally in the stomach backs up into the esophagus. This condition is also called "gastroesophageal reflux disease," or GERD.

The symptoms of acid reflux include:

- Burning in the chest (heartburn)

- Burning or acid taste in the throat

- Stomach or chest pain

- Difficulty in swallowing

- Raspy voice or a sore throat

- Unexplained cough (not in laryngectomees unless their voice prosthesis leaks)

- In laryngectomees: granulation tissue forms around the voice prosthesis, short voice prosthesis device life, voice problems

Measures to reduce and prevent acid reflux include:

- Losing weight (in those who are overweight)

- Reducing stress and practicing relaxation techniques

- Avoiding foods that worsen symptoms (e.g., coffee, chocolate, alcohol, peppermint, and fatty foods)

- Stopping smoking and passive exposure to smoke

- Eating small amounts of food several times a day, rather than large meals

- Sitting upright when eating and staying upright thirty to sixty minutes later

- Avoiding lying down for three hours after a meal

- Elevating the head of the bed by 6-8 inches (by putting blocks of wood under two legs of the bed or a wedge under the mattress) or by using pillows to elevate the upper portion of the body by at least about 45 degrees

- Taking a medication that reduces the production of stomach acids, as prescribed by one's physician

- When bending down, bend the knees rather than bend the upper body

Medications for the treatment of acid reflux. There are three major types of medication that can help reduce acid reflux symptoms: antacids, histamine H2-receptor antagonists (also known as H2 blockers), and proton pump inhibitors. These drug classes work in different ways by reducing or blocking stomach acid.

Liquid antacids are generally more active than tablets, and more active if taken after a meal or before going to bed, but they work only for a short time. H2 blockers (e.g., Pepcid, Tagamet, Zantac) work by reducing the amount of acid produced by the stomach. They last longer than antacids and can relieve mild symptoms. Most H2 blockers can be bought without a prescription.

Proton pump inhibitors (e.g., Prilosec, Nexium, Prevacid, Aciphex) are the most effective medicines in treating GERD and stopping the production of stomach acid. Some of these medicines are sold without a prescription. They may reduce the absorption of calcium. Monitoring the serum calcium levels is important; individuals with low calcium levels may need to take calcium supplements.

It is advisable to see a physician if the GERD symptoms are severe or last a long time and are difficult to control.

Speaking when eating and after laryngectomy

Laryngectomees who speak through a tracheoesophageal voice prosthesis have difficulties in speaking when they swallow. This is especially challenging during the time it takes the food or liquids to pass by the esophageal TEP site. Speaking during that time is either impossible or sounds "bubbly." This is because the air introduced into the esophagus through the voice prosthesis has to travel through the food or liquids. Unfortunately it takes the food much longer to go through the esophagus, in someone who has had a flap to replace the pharynx. This is because the flap has no peristalsis (contraction and relaxation), the food goes down mainly due to gravity.

It is therefore important to eat slowly, mix the food with liquids while chewing and allow the food to pass through the TEP area before trying to speak. Over time, laryngectomees can learn how much time is needed for food to pass through the esophagus to allow speech. It is helpful to drink before attempting to speak after eating.

There are eating and swallowing exercises that a speech and language pathologist (SLP) can teach a laryngectomee that may assist them in relearning how to swallow without difficulties.

Swallowing difficulties

Most laryngectomees experience problems with swallowing (dysphagia) immediately after their surgery. Because swallowing involves the coordination between more than twenty muscles and several nerves, damage to any part of the system by surgery or radiation can produce swallowing difficulties. The majority of laryngectomees relearn how to swallow with minimal problems. Some may only need to make minor adjustments in eating such as taking smaller bites, chewing more thoroughly, and drinking more liquids while eating. Some experience significant swallowing difficulties and require assistance in learning how to improve their ability to swallow by working with a SLP who specializes in swallowing disorders.

Swallowing functions change after a laryngectomy and can be further complicated by radiation and chemotherapy. The incidence of swallowing difficulty and food obstruction can be as high as fifty percent of patients, and if not addressed, can lead to malnutrition. Most difficulties with swallowing are noticed after discharge from the hospital. They can occur when attempting to eat too fast and not chewing well. They can also happen after trauma to the upper esophagus by ingesting a sharp piece of food or drinking very hot liquid. These can cause swelling which may last a day or two. (I describe my personal experiences with eating in my book "My Voice" in Chapter 20 entitled Eating.)

Swallowing problems (or dysphagia) are common after total laryngectomy. The problems may be temporary or long term. Risks of swallowing problems include poor nutritional status, limitations in social situations and diminished quality of life.

Patients experience difficulties in swallowing as a result of:

- Abnormal function of the pharyngeal muscles (dysmotility)

- Cricopharyngeal dysfunction of the the cricoid cartilage and the pharynx

- Reduced strength of the movements of the base of the tongue

- Development of a fold of mucous membrane or scar tissue at the tongue base called "pseudoepiglottis". Food can collect between the pseudoepiglottis and the tongue base

- Difficulty with tongue movements, chewing, and food propulsion in the pharynx because of removal of the hyoid bone and other structural changes

- A stricture within the pharynx or esophagus may decrease food passage leading to its collection

- Development of a pouch (diverticulum) in the pharyngoesophageal wall that can collect fluid and food resulting in the complaint of food "sticking" in the upper esophagus

Laryngectomees are usually not allowed to swallow food immediately after surgery and must be fed through a feeding tube for two to three weeks. The tube is inserted into the stomach through the nose, mouth or the tracheo-esophageal puncture and liquid nourishment is supplied through the tube. This practice, however, is slowly changing; there is increasing evidence that in standard surgeries, oral intake can start with clear liquids as soon as 24 hours after surgery. This may also help with swallowing as the muscles involved will continue to be used.

Following an episode of food obstruction in the upper esophagus swallowing may be difficult for a day or two. This is probably because of the local swelling in the back of the throat; normally, this will disappear with time.

Ways to avoid such episodes:

- Eating slowly and patiently

- Taking small bites of food and chewing very well

- Swallowing a small amount of food at a time and always mixing it with liquid in the mouth before swallowing. Warm liquid makes it easier to swallow.

- Flushing the food with more liquids as needed (warm liquids may work better for some individuals in flushing down the food).

- Avoiding food that is sticky or hard to chew. One needs to find out for him/her self what food is easier to ingest. Some foods are easy to swallow (e.g., toasted or dry bread, yogurt, and bananas) and others tend to be sticky (e.g., unpeeled apples, lettuce and other leafy vegetables, and steak).

Swallowing problems may improve over time. However, dilatation of the esophagus may be needed if the narrowing is permanent. The extent of the narrowing can be evaluated by a swallow test. Dilatation is usually done by an otolaryngologist or a gastroenterologist (see **Dilation of the esophagus,** page 96.)

Tests used for the evaluation of swallowing difficulty

There are five major tests that can be used for the evaluation of swallowing difficulties:

- Barium swallow radiography

- Videofluoroscopy (motion X-ray study)

- Upper endoscopic evaluation of swallowing

- Fiberoptic nasopharyngeal laryngoscopy

- Esophageal manometry (measures esophagus muscle contractions)

The specific test is chosen according to the clinical condition.

Videofluoroscopy which is usually the first test done to most patients, records swallowing during fluoroscopy. It allows accurate visualization and study of the sequence of events which make up a swallow; it is limited to the cervical esophagus. The video, taken from both the front and the side, can be viewed at much slower speeds to enable accurate study. This helps identify abnormal movement of food, such as aspiration, pooling, movement of anatomic structures, muscle activities, and exact oral and pharyngeal transit times. The effects of various barium consistencies and positions can be tested. Thick or solid food boluses can be used for patients who complain of solid food dysphagia.

Narrowing of the esophagus and swallowing problems

A stricture of the esophagus is a narrowing along the pharyngo-esophagus that blocks or inhibits the ease of food passage, resulting in the esophagus having an hour-glass configuration.

Strictures after laryngectomy can be due to the effects of radiation and the tightness of the surgical closure and can also develop gradually as scarring forms.

Interventions that can help the patient include:

- Dietary and postural changes

- Myotomy (cutting the muscle)

- Dilatation (see below)

The free flap that is sometimes used to replace the larynx has no peristalsis, making swallowing even more difficult. After surgery in such cases the food descends to the stomach mostly by gravity. The time for the food to reach the stomach varies between individuals and ranges from 5 to 10 seconds.

Chewing the food well and mixing it with liquid in the mouth prior to swallowing is helpful, as is swallowing only small amounts of food each time, and waiting for it to go down. Drinking liquids between solid foods is helpful in flushing down the food. Eating takes longer; one must learn to be patient and take all the time needed to finish the meal.

The swelling immediately after surgery tends to decrease over time which reduces the narrowing of the esophagus and ultimately makes swallowing easier. This is good to remember because there is always hope that swallowing will improve within the first few months after surgery. However, if this does not occur dilatation of the esophagus is one therapeutic option.

Dilatation of the esophagus

Narrowing of the esophagus is a very common consequence of laryngectomy; dilatation of the narrow esophagus is often needed to reopen it. The procedure usually needs to be repeated and the frequency of this procedure varies among individuals. In some people this is a lifelong requirement and in others the esophagus may stay open after a few dilatations. The procedure requires sedation or anesthesia because it is painful. A series of dilators with greater diameter are introduced into the esophagus to dilate it slowly. While the process breaks down the fibrosis, the condition may return after a while.

Sometimes a balloon rather than a long dilator is used to dilate a local stricture. Another method that may help is the use of topical and injectable steroids in the esophagus. Although dilation is done by an otolaryngologist or a gastroenterologist, in some cases it can be accomplished by the patient at home. In difficult cases, surgery may be needed to remove the stricture or replace the narrow section with a graft.

Because dilation breaks down fibrosis, the pain generated by the procedure may last for a while. Taking pain medication can ease the discomfort. (See **Pain management,** page 101)

Use of Botox®

Botox® is a pharmaceutical preparation of toxin A which is produced by *Clostridium botulinum*, an anaerobic bacteria that causes botulism, a muscle paralysis illness. The botulinum toxin causes partial paralysis of muscles by acting on their presynaptic cholinergic nerve fibers through the prevention of the release of acetylcholine at the neuromuscular junction. In small quantities it can be used to temporarily paralyze muscles for three to four months. It is used to control muscle spasms, excessive blinking, and for cosmetic treatment of wrinkles. Infrequent side effects are generalized muscle weakness and rarely even death. Botox® injection has become the treatment of choice for selected individuals to improve swallowing and tracheo-esophageal speech after laryngectomy.

For laryngectomees, injections of Botox® has been used to reduce the hypertonicity and spasm of the vibrating segment, resulting in an esophageal or trachea-esophageal voice that requires less effort to produce. However, it is only effective for overactive muscles and may require the injection of relatively large doses into the spastic muscles. It can also be used to relax muscle tightness in the lower jaw when one experiences difficulties in swallowing. It cannot help conditions that are not due to muscle spasms such as esophageal diverticula, strictures due to fibrosis after radiation, and scars and narrowing after surgery.

A constrictor muscle hypertonicity or pharyngoesophageal spasm (PES) is a common cause for tracheo-esophageal speech failure following laryngectomy. Constrictor muscle hypertonicity can increase peak intra-esophageal pressure during speaking, thus interfering with fluent speech. It may also disturb swallowing by interfering with the pharyngeal transit of food and liquids.

Botox® injection can be carried out by otolaryngologists in the clinic. The injection can be done percutaneously or through an esophago-gastro-duodenoscope. The percutaneous injection into the pharyngeal constrictor muscles along one side of the newly formed pharynx (neopharynx) is done just above and to the side of the stoma.

An injection through an esophago-gastro-duodenoscope can be performed whenever a percutaneous injection is not feasible. This method is used in patients with severe post-radiation fibrosis, disruption of the cervical anatomy, and anxiety or inability to withstand a percutaneous injection. This method allows direct visualization and greater precision. The injection into the PES segment is often done by a gastroenterologist and is followed by gentle expansion by balloon massage to facilitate uniform distribution of the Botox®.

Pharyngo-cutaneous fistula

A pharyngo-cutaneous fistula is an abnormal connection between the pharyngeal mucosa to the skin. Typically a salivary leak develops from the pharyngeal area to the skin, indicating a breakdown of the pharyngeal surgical suture line. It is the most common complication after laryngectomy and usually occurs seven to ten days after the operation. Previous radiation is a risk factor. Oral feeding is withheld until the fistula heals by itself or is surgically repaired.

The closure of the fistula can be evaluated by a "dye test" (such as ingestion of methylene blue which appears in the skin if the fistula is unobstructed) and/or by radiograhic contrast studies.

Smelling after laryngectomy

Laryngectomees may experience difficulties with their sense of smell. This is despite the fact that regular laryngectomy surgery does not involve nerves related to the sense of smell and the sense of smell, or olfaction, remains intact. What has changed, however, is the pathway of airflow during respiration. Before a laryngectomy, air flows into the lungs through the nose and mouth. This movement of air through the nose allows for scents and aromas to be detected as they come in contact with the nerve endings in the nose responsible for the sense of smell.

After a laryngectomy, however, there is no longer an active air flow through the nose. This can be perceived as a loss of smell. The "polite yawn technique" can help laryngectomees regain their capacity to smell. This method is known as the "polite yawn technique" because the movements involved are similar to those used when one attempt to yawn with a closed mouth. Swift, downward movement of the lower jaw and tongue, while keeping the lips closed, will create a subtle vacuum, drawing air into the nasal passages and enabling the detection of any scent through the new airflow. With practice, it is possible to achieve the same vacuum using more subtle (but effective) tongue movements.

CHAPTER 12:

Medical issues after radiation and surgery: pain management, cancer spread, hypothyroidism, and prevention of medical errors

This section describes a variety of medical issues affecting laryngectomees.

Hypertension is discussed in page 28 and **Lymphedema** in page 37.

Pain management

Many cancer patients and survivors complain of pain. Pain can be one of the important signs of cancer and may even lead to its diagnosis. Thus, it should not be ignored and should be a sign to seek medical care. The pain associated with cancer can vary in intensity and quality. It can be constant, intermittent, mild, moderate or severe. It can also be aching, dull, or sharp.

The pain can be caused by a tumor pressing or growing into and destroying nearby tissues. As the tumor increases in size, it may cause pain by putting pressure on nerves, bones or other structures. Cancer of the head and neck can also erode the mucosa and expose it to saliva and mouth bacteria. Cancer that has spread or recurred is even more likely to cause pain.

Pain can result also from treatments for cancer. Chemotherapy, radiation and surgery are all potential sources of pain. Chemotherapy can cause diarrhea, mouth sores, and nerve damage. Radiation of the head and neck may cause painful and burning sensations to the skin and mouth, muscle stiffness and nerve damage. Surgery also can be painful, may leave deformities and/or scars that take time to improve.

Cancer pain can be treated by various methods. Eliminating the source of the pain through radiation, chemotherapy, or surgery is best, if possible. However, if not possible, other treatments include oral medication, nerve blocks, acupuncture, acupressure, massage, physical therapy, meditation, relaxation, and even humor. Specialists in pain management can offer these treatments.

Pain medication can be administered as a tablet, dissolvable tablet, intravenously, intramuscularly, rectally or through a skin patch. Medication includes: analgesics (e.g., aspirin, acetaminophen), nonsteroidal anti-inflammatory drugs (e.g., ibuprofen), weak (e.g., codeine) and strong (e.g., morphine, oxycodone, hydromorphone, fentanyl, methadone) opioids.

Sometimes patients do not receive adequate treatment for cancer pain. The reasons for this include doctors' reluctance to inquire about pain or offer treatments, patients' reluctance to speak about their pain, fear of addiction to medication, and fear of side effects.

Treating pain can both increase patients' well-being, as well as ease the hardship imposed on their caregivers. Patients should be encouraged to talk to their health care providers about their pain and seek treatment. Evaluation by a pain management specialist can be very helpful; all major cancer centers have pain management programs.

Symptoms and signs of recurrent or new head and neck cancer

Most individuals with head and neck cancer receive medical and surgical treatment that removes and eradicates the cancer. However, there is always the possibility that the cancer may recur; vigilance is needed to detect recurrence or possibly new primary tumors. It is therefore very important to be aware of the signs of laryngeal and other types of head and neck cancer so that they can be detected at an early stage.

Signs and symptoms of head and neck cancer include:

- Bloody sputum

- Bleeding from the nose, throat, mouth

- Lumps on or outside the neck

- Lumps or white, red or dark patches inside the mouth

- Abnormal-sounding or difficult breathing

- Chronic cough

- Changes in voice (including hoarseness)

- Neck pain or swelling

- Difficulty in chewing, swallowing or moving the tongue

- Thickening of the cheek(s)

- Pain around the teeth, or loosening of the teeth

- A sore in the mouth that doesn't heal or increases in size

- Numbness of the tongue or elsewhere in the mouth

- Persistent mouth, throat or ear pain

- Bad breath

- Weight loss

Individuals with these symptoms should be examined by their otolaryngologists as soon as possible.

Head and neck cancer spread

Laryngeal cancer like other head and neck cancers, can spread to the lungs and the liver. The risk of spread is higher in larger tumors and in tumors that had been recognized late. The greater risk of spread is in the first five years and especially in the first two years after the cancer appears. If the local lymph glands do not reveal cancer the risk is lower.

Individuals who had cancer at one time may be more likely to develop another type of malignancy not related to their head and neck cancer. As people age, they often develop other medical problems that require care, for example, hypertension and diabetes. It is therefore imperative to receive adequate nutrition, take care of one's dental (See **Dental issues,** page 117), physical and mental health, be under good medical care and be examined on a regular basis (See **Follow-up by family physician, internist and medical specialists,** Page 112). Of course, head and neck cancer survivors, like everyone else, need to watch for all types of cancers. These are relatively easy to diagnose by regular examination and include breast, cervix, prostate, colon, and skin cancer.

Low thyroid hormone (hypothyroidism) and its treatment

Most laryngectomees develop low levels of the thyroid hormone (hypothyroidism). This is due to the effects of radiation and the removal of part or all of the thyroid gland during laryngectomy surgery.

The symptoms of hypothyroidism vary; some individuals have no symptoms while others have dramatic or, rarely, life-threatening symptoms. The symptoms of hypothyroidism are nonspecific and mimic many normal changes of aging.

General symptoms — The thyroid hormone stimulates the body's metabolism. Most symptoms of hypothyroidism are due to the slowing of metabolic processes. Systemic symptoms include fatigue, sluggishness, weight gain, and intolerance to cold temperatures.

Skin — Decreased sweating, dry and thick skin, coarse or thin hair, disappearance of eyebrows, and brittle nails.

Eyes — Mild swelling around the eyes

Cardiovascular system — Slowing of the heart rate and weakening of the contractions, decreasing its overall function. These can cause fatigue and shortness of breath with exercise. Hypothyroidism can also cause mild hypertension and raise cholesterol levels.

Respiratory system — Respiratory muscles can weaken, and lung function can decrease. Symptoms include fatigue, shortness of breath with exercise, and decreased ability to exercise. Hypothyroidism may lead to swelling of the tongue, hoarse voice, and sleep apnea (not in laryngectomees).

Gastrointestinal system — Slowing of the digestive tract actions, causing constipation

Reproductive system — Menstrual cycle irregularities, ranging from absent or infrequent periods to very frequent and heavy periods

Thyroid deficiency can be corrected by taking synthetic thyroid hormone (Thyroxine). This medicine should be taken on an empty stomach with a full glass of water thirty minutes before eating, preferably before breakfast or at a similar time of day. This is because food containing high fat (e.g., eggs, bacon, toast, hash brown potatoes, and milk) can decrease thyroxine absorption by forty percent.

Several formulations of synthetic thyroxine are available, but there has been considerable controversy if they are similar in efficacy. In 2004 the FDA approved a generic substitute for branded levothyroxine products. The American Thyroid Association, Endocrine Society, and the American Association of Clinical Endocrinologists objected to this decision, recommending that patients remain on the same brand. If patients must switch brands or use a generic substitute, serum thyroid stimulating hormone (TSH) should be checked six weeks later.

Because there may be subtle differences between synthetic thyroxine formulations, it is better to stay with one formulation when possible. If the preparation must be changed, follow-up monitoring of TSH and sometimes free thyroxine (T4) serum levels should be done to determine if dose adjustments are necessary.

After starting therapy, the patient should be reevaluated and serum TSH should be measured in three to six weeks, and the dose adjusted if needed. Symptoms of hypothyroidism generally begin to resolve after two to three weeks of replacement therapy and may take at least six weeks to dissipate.

A thyroxine dose can be increased in three weeks in those who continue to have symptoms and who have a high serum TSH concentration. It takes about six weeks before a steady hormone state is achieved after therapy is initiated or the dose is changed.

This process of increasing the dose of hormone every three to six weeks is continued, based upon periodic measurements of TSH until it returns to normal (from approximately 0.5 to 5.0 mU/L). Once this is achieved, periodic monitoring is needed.

After identification of the proper maintenance dose, the patient should be examined and serum TSH measured once a year (or more often if there is an abnormal result or a change in the patient's condition). Dose adjustment may be needed as patients age or have a weight change.

Preventing medical and surgical errors

Medical and surgical mistakes are very common. They increase malpractice lawsuits, the cost of medical care, patients' hospital stays, and morbidity and mortality.

A manuscript describing my personal experiences facing medical and surgical errors in my care was published in Disabled-World.com at
http://www.disabled-world.com/disability/publications/neck-cancer-patient.php

The best way of preventing errors is for the patient to be his or her own advocate or have a family member or friend serve as one's advocate.

Medical errors can be reduced by:

- Being informed and not hesitating to challenge and ask for explanations

- Becoming an "expert" in one's medical issues

- Having a family or friends remain in the hospital

- Getting a second opinion

- Educating medical providers about one's condition and needs (prior to and after surgery)

The occurrence of errors weakens patients trust in their health care providers. Admission and acceptance of responsibility by medical providers can bridge the gap between them and the patient and can reestablish lost confidence. When such a dialogue is established, more details about the circumstances leading to the mistake can be learned thus helping to prevent similar errors. Open discussion can assure patients that their providers are taking the mater seriously and that steps will be taken to make their hospital stays safer.

Not discussing mistakes with the patient and family increases their anxiety, frustration and anger, thus interfering with their recovery. And of course, such anger may also lead to malpractice suits.

Greater vigilance by the medical community can reduce errors. Obviously medical errors should be prevented as much as humanly possible; ignoring them can only lead to their repetition. Institutional policies should support and encourage healthcare professionals to disclose adverse events. Increased openness and honesty following adverse events can improve provider-patient relationships. There are important preventive steps that can be implemented by every institution and medical office. Educating the patient and their caregivers about the patient's condition and treatment plan is of utmost importance. Medical professionals can safeguard and prevent mistakes when they see deviations from the planned therapy.

These steps by the medical establishment can prevent medical errors:

- Implement better and uniform medical training

- Adhere to well established standards of care

- Perform regular records review to detect and correct medical errors

- Employ only well educated and trained medical staff

- Counsel, reprimand, and educate staff members who make errors and dismiss those who continue to err

- Develop and meticulously follow algorithms (specific sets of instructions for procedures), establish protocols and bedside checklists for all interventions

- Increase supervision and communication among health care providers

- Investigate all errors and take action to prevent them

- Educate and inform the patient and his/her caregivers about the patient's condition and treatment plans

- Have a family member and or friend serve as a patient advocate to ensure the appropriateness of the management

- Respond to patients' and family complaints, admit responsibility when appropriate, discuss these with the family and staff and take action to prevent the error(s)

CHAPTER 13:

Preventive care: follow-up, avoiding smoking, and vaccination

Preventive medical and dental care is essential for patients with cancer. Many individuals with cancer neglect to attend to other important medical problems and focus exclusively on their cancer. Neglecting other medical issues can lead to serious consequences that may influence well-being and longevity.

The most important preventive measures for laryngectomees and head and neck cancer patients include:

- Proper dental care

- Routine examinations by family physician

- Routine follow-up by an otolaryngologist

- Appropriate vaccinations

- Stop smoking

- Using proper techniques (e.g., using sterile water for stoma irrigation)

- Maintaining adequate nutrition

Routine dental follow-up and dental preventive care are discussed in Chapter 14 (page 117).

Using proper techniques for stoma care is presented in Chapter 8 (page 59).

Adequate nutrition is discussed in Chapter 11 (page 85).

Follow-up by family physician, internist and medical specialists

Continual medical follow-up by specialists, including the otolaryngologist, radiation oncologist (for those who got radiation treatment), and oncologist (for those who received chemotherapy), is crucial. As time passes from the initial diagnosis, treatment and surgery, follow-up occurs with less frequency. Most otolaryngologists recommend monthly follow-up examination in the first year after diagnosis and or surgery and less often afterwards, depending on the patient's condition. Patients should be encouraged to contact their physician whenever new symptoms arise.

Regular checkups ensure that any changes in health are noted and that whenever a new problem emerges it is addressed and treated. The clinician will perform a careful examination to detect cancer recurrence. Checkups include a general examination of the entire body and specific examination of the neck, throat and stoma. Examination of the upper airway is performed using an endoscope or indirect visualization with a small, long-handled mirror to check for abnormal areas. Radiological and other studies may also be performed as needed.

It is also very important to be followed by an internist or family physician, as well as dentist, to address other medical and dental issues.

Influenza vaccination

It is important for laryngectomees to be vaccinated for influenza regardless of age. Influenza can be more difficult to manage and vaccination is an important preventive tool.

There are two types of influenza vaccine: an injection one that is adequate for all ages and an inhalation one (live virus) only given to individuals younger than fifty years who are not immune-compromised.

Available vaccines include:

1. The "flu shot" - an inactivated vaccine (containing killed virus) given by a needle, usually in the arm. The flu shot is approved for persons older than six months, including healthy individuals and those with chronic medical conditions.

2. The nasal-spray flu vaccine - a vaccine made with live, weakened flu viruses that do not cause the flu (sometimes called LAIV for "live attenuated influenza vaccine" or FluMist®). LAIV is approved for use in healthy individuals ages 2-49 years (with the exception of pregnant women).

A new vaccine for influenza is prepared for every new season. While the exact strains that cause influenza are unpredictable, it is likely that strains that caused the illness at other parts of the world will also cause illness in the U.S. It is best to consult one's physician prior to vaccination to ensure that there is no reason why one should not be vaccinated (such as egg allergy).

The best way to diagnose Influenza is a rapid test of nasal secretions by one of the diagnostic kits. Because laryngectomees have no connection between the nose and the lungs, it is advisable to test nasal secretions in addition to tracheal sputum (using a kit that was approved for sputum testing).

Information about these tests can be found in the Center of Disease Control website (http://www.cdc.gov/flu/professionals/diagnosis/rapidlab.htm).

One "advantage" of being a laryngecomee is that one generally gets fewer infections caused by respiratory tract viruses. This is because "cold" viruses generally first infect the nose and throat; from there they travel to the rest of the body, including the lungs. Because laryngectomees do not breathe through their noses, cold viruses are less likely to infect them.

It is still important for laryngectomees to receive yearly immunization for influenza viruses, to wear a Heat and Moisture Exchanger (HME) device to filter the air that gets into the lungs, and to wash their hands well before touching the stoma or the HME or before eating. The Atos (Provox) Micron HME with electrostatic filter is designed to filtrate potential pathogens and to reduce susceptibility to respiratory infections.

The influenza virus is capable of spreading by touching objects. Laryngectomees who use a voice prosthesis and need to press their HME to speak may be at increased risk of introducing the virus directly to their lungs. Washing hands or using a skin cleanser can prevent the spread of the virus.

Vaccination against the pneumococcal bacteria

It is advisable that laryngectomees and other neck breathers get vaccinated against the pneumococcus bacteria which is one of the major causes of pneumonia. In the United States there are two types of vaccines against the pneumococcal bacteria: the pneumococcal conjugate vaccine (Prevnar 13 or PCV13) and the pneumococcal polysaccharaide vaccine - a 23-valent pneumococcal polysaccharide vaccine (Pneumovax or PPV23).

One should consult their physician about receiving the pneumococcal vaccination.

The Center for Disease Control publishes the current guidelines at: http://www.cdc.gov/vaccines/

Avoiding smoking and alcohol

Individuals with head and neck cancer should receive counseling about the importance of smoking cessation. In addition to smoking being a major risk factor for head and neck cancer, the risk of cancer is further enhanced by alcohol consumption. Smoking can also influence cancer prognosis. Patients with laryngeal cancer who continue to smoke and drink are less likely to be cured and are more likely to develop a second tumor. When smoking is continued both during and after radiation therapy, it can increase the severity and duration of mucosal reactions, worsen the dry mouth (xerostomia), and compromise the patient outcome.

Smoking tobacco and drinking alcohol also decrease the effectiveness of treatment for laryngeal cancer. Patients who continue to smoke while receiving radiation therapy have a lower long-term survival rate than those who do not smoke.

CHAPTER 14:

Dental Issues and hyperbaric oxygen therapy

Dental issues can be challenging for laryngectomees, mainly because of the long term effects of radiation therapy. Maintenance of good dental hygiene can prevent many problems.

Dental Issues

Dental problems are common after exposure of the head and neck to radiation therapy.

Radiation affects include:

- Reduced blood supply to the maxillary and mandibular bones

- Reduced production and changes in the chemical composition of saliva

- Changes in the bacteria that colonize the mouth

Because of these changes dental caries, soreness, and gingival and periodontal inflammation can be particularly problematic. These can be lessened by good mouth and teeth care, i.e., by cleaning, flushing, and using fluorinated toothpaste after each meal when possible. Using a special fluorinated preparation with which to gargle or apply on the gum helps in preventing dental carries. Keeping well hydrated and using saliva substitute when needed are also important.

It is advisable that patients receiving radiation therapy to the head and neck visit their dentist for a thorough oral examination several weeks prior to initiation of the treatment and be examined on a regular annual or semiannual basis throughout life. Getting regular dental cleaning is also important.

Because radiation treatment alters the blood supply to the maxillary and mandibular bones patients may be at risk of developing bone necrosis (**osteoradionecrosis**) at those sites. Tooth extraction and dental disease in irradiated areas can lead to the development of osteoradionecrosis. Patients should inform their dentist about their radiation treatment prior to these procedures. Osteoradionecrosis may be prevented by administration of a series of hyperbaric oxygen therapy (see below) before and after extraction or dental surgery. This is recommended if the involved tooth is in an area that had been exposed to a high dose of radiation. Consulting the radiation oncologist who delivered the radiation treatment can be helpful in determining if this is necessary.

Dental prophylaxis can reduce the risk of dental problems leading to bone necrosis. Special fluoride treatments may help to prevent dental problems, along with brushing, flossing, and having one's teeth cleaned regularly.

A home care dental lifelong routine is recommended:

- Flossing each tooth and brushing with toothpaste after each meal

- Brushing the tongue with a tongue brush or a soft bristled toothbrush once a day

- Rinsing with a baking soda rinse daily. Baking soda helps neutralize the mouth. The rinse is made of one teaspoon of baking soda added to 12 oz. of water. The baking soda rinse can be used throughout the day.

- Using fluoride in fluoride carriers once a day. These are commercially available and are also custom made by dentists. They are applied over the teeth for ten minutes. One should not rinse, drink, or eat for thirty minutes after fluoride application.

Stomach acid reflux is also very common after head and neck surgery, especially in individuals who have had partial or complete laryngectomy (see **Symptoms and treatment of stomach acid reflux,** page 89). This can also cause dental erosion (especially of the lower jaw) and, ultimately teeth loss.

These ill effects can be reduced by:

- Taking acid reducing medication

- Eating small amounts of food and liquid each time

- Not lying down right after eating

- When lying down, elevate the upper part of body with a pillow to 45 degrees

Hyperbaric oxygen therapy

Hyperbaric oxygen (HBO) therapy involves breathing pure oxygen in a pressurized room. HBO therapy is a well-established treatment for decompression sickness (a hazard of scuba diving) and can be used to prevent osteoradionecrosis.

HBO is used to treat a wide range of medical conditions including bubbles of air in the blood vessels (arterial gas embolism), decompression sickness, carbon monoxide poisoning, a wound that won't heal, a crush injury, gangrene, skin or bone infection causing tissue death (such a osteoradionecrosis), radiation injuries, burns, skin grafts or skin flaps at risk of tissue death, and severe anemia.

In an HBO therapy chamber, the air pressure is raised up to three times higher than normal air pressure. Under these conditions, the lungs can gather much more oxygen than is possible when breathing pure oxygen at normal air pressure.

The blood carries this oxygen throughout the body, stimulating the release of chemicals called "growth factors" and stem cells that promote healing. When tissue is injured, it requires even more oxygen to survive. HBO therapy increases the amount of oxygen in the blood and can temporarily restore normal levels of blood gases and tissue function. These promote healing and the ability of the tissues to fight infection.

HBO therapy is generally safe and complications are rare. These can include: temporary nearsightedness (myopia), middle ear and inner ear injuries (including leaking fluid and eardrum rupture due to increased air pressure), organ damage caused by air pressure changes (barotrauma), and seizures as a result of oxygen toxicity.

Pure oxygen can cause a fire if there is a source of ignition, such as a spark or flame. It is therefore forbidden to take items that could ignite a fire (e.g., lighters or battery powered devices) into the HBO therapy room.

HBO therapy can be performed as an outpatient procedure and does not require hospitalization. Hospitalized patients may need to be transported to and from the HBO therapy site if it is an outside facility.

Treatment can be performed in one of two settings:

- **A unit designed for one person** in an individual (monoplace) unit, while the patient lies down on a padded table that slides into a clear plastic tube.

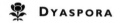 **DYASPORA**

Joanne Hyppolite

When you are in Haiti they call you *Dyaspora*. This word, which connotes both connection and disconnection, accurately describes your condition as a Haitian American. Disconnected from the physical landscape of the homeland, you don't grow up with a mango tree in your yard, you don't suck *kenèps* in the summer, or sit in the dark listening to stories of *Konpè* Bouki and Malis. The bleat of *vaksins* or the beating of a *Yanvalou* on *Rada* drums are neither in the background or the foreground of your life. Your French is non-existent. Haiti is not where you live.

Your house in Boston is your island. As the only Haitian family on the hillside street you grow up on, it represents Haiti to you. It was where your *granmè* refused to learn English, where goods like ripe mangoes, plantains, *djondjon*, and hard white blobs of mints come to you in boxes through the mail. At your communion and birthday parties, all of Boston Haiti seems to gather in your house to eat *griyo* and sip *kremas*. It takes forever for you to kiss every cheek, some of them heavy with face powder, some of them damp with perspiration, some of them with scratchy face hair, and some of them giving you a perfume head-rush as you swoop in. You are grateful for every smooth, dry cheek you encounter. In your house, the dreaded

7

matinèt which your parents imported from Haiti just to keep you, your brother, and your sister in line sits threateningly on top of the wardrobe. It is where your mother's *andeyò Kreyòl* accent and your father's *lavil* French accent make sometimes beautiful, sometimes terrible music together. On Sundays in your house, "Dominika-anik-anik" floats from the speakers of the record player early in the morning and you are made to put on one of your frilly dresses, your matching lace-edged socks, and black shoes. Your mother ties long ribbons into a bow at the root of each braid. She warns you, your brother and your sister to "respect your heads" as you drive to St. Angela's, never missing a Sunday service in fourteen years. In your island house, everyone has two names. The name they were given and the nickname they have been granted so that your mother is Gisou, your father is Popo, your brother is Claudy, your sister is Tinou, you are Jojo, and your grandmother is Manchoun. Every day your mother serves rice and beans and you methodically pick out all the beans because you don't like *pwa*. You think they are ugly and why does all the rice have to have beans anyway? Even with the white rice or the *mayi moulen*, your mother makes *sòs pwa*— bean sauce. You develop the idea that Haitians are obsessed with beans. In your house there is a mortar and a pestle as well as five pictures of Jesus, your parents drink Café Bustelo every morning, your father wears *gwayabèl* shirts and smokes cigarettes, and you are beaten when you don't get good grades at school. You learn about the infidelities of husbands from conversations your aunts have. You are dragged to Haitian plays, Haitian *bals*, and Haitian concerts where in spite of yourself *konpa* rhythms make you sway. You know the names of Haitian presidents and military leaders because political discussions inevitably erupt whenever there are more than three Haitian men together in the same place. Every time you are sick, your mother rubs you down with a foul-smelling liquid that she keeps in an old Barbancourt rum bottle under her bed. You splash yourself with Bien-être after every bath. Your parents speak to you in *Kreyòl*, you respond in English, and somehow this works and feels natural. But when your mother speaks English, things seem to go wrong. She makes no distinction between he and she, and you become the pronoun police. Every day you get a visit from some *matant* or *monnonk* or *kouzen* who is also a *marenn* or *parenn* of someone in the house. In your house, your grandmother has a porcelain *kivèt* she keeps under her bed to relieve herself at night. You pore over photograph albums where there are pictures of you going to school in Haiti, in the yard in Haiti, under the white Christmas tree in Haiti, and you marvel because you do not remember anything that you see. You do not remember Haiti because you left there too young but it does not matter because it is as if Haiti has lassoed your house with an invisible rope.

Outside of your house, you are forced to sink or swim in American waters. For you this means an Irish-Catholic school and a Black-American neighborhood. The school is a choice made by your parents who strongly believe in a private Catholic education anyway, not paying any mind to the busing crisis that is raging in the city. The choice of neighborhood is a condition of the reality of living here in this city with its racially segregated neighborhoods. Before you lived here, white people owned this hillside street. After you and others who looked like you came, they gradually disappeared to other places, leaving you this place and calling it bad because you and others like you live there now. As any *dyaspora* child knows, Haitian parents are not familiar with these waters. They say things to you like, "In Haiti we never treated white people badly." They don't know about racism. They don't know about the latest styles and fashions and give your brother hell every time he sneaks out to a friend's house and gets his hair cut into a shag, a high-top, a fade.

They don't know that the ribbons in your hair, the gold loops in your ears, and the lace that edges your socks alert other children to your difference. So you wait until you get to school before taking them all off and out and you put them back on at the end of your street where the bus drops you off. Outside your house, things are black and white. You are black and white. Especially in your school where neither you nor any of the few other Haitian girls in your class are invited to the birthday parties of the white kids in your class. You cleave to these other Haitian girls out of something that begins as solidarity but becomes a lifetime of friendship. You make green hats in art class every St. Patrick's day and watch Irish step-dancing shows year after year after year. You discover books and reading and this is what you do when you take the bus home, just you and your white schoolmates. You lose your accent. You study about the Indians in social studies but you do not study about Black Americans except in music class where you are forced to sing Negro spirituals as a concession to your presence. They don't know anything about Toussaint Louverture or Jean-Jacques Dessalines.

In your neighborhood when you tell people you are from Haiti, they ask politely, "Where's that?" You explain and because you seem okay to them, Haiti is okay to them. They shout "Hi, Grunny!" whenever they see your grandmother on the stoop and sometimes you translate a sentence or two between them. In their houses, you eat sweet potato pie and nod because you have that too, it's made a little different and you call it *pen patat* but it's the same taste after all. From the girls on the street you learn to jump double-dutch, you learn to dance the puppet and the white boy. You see a woman preacher for the first time in your life at their church. You wonder where down South is because that is where most of the boys and girls on your block go for vacations. You learn about boys and sex through these girls because these two subjects are not allowed in your island/house. You keep your street friends separate from your school friends and this is how it works and you are used to it. You get so you can jump between worlds with the same ease that you slide on your nightgown every evening.

Then when you get to high school, things change. People in your high school and your neighborhood look at you and say, "You are Haitian?" and from the surprise in their voice you realize that they know where Haiti is now. They think they know what Haiti is now. Haiti is the boat people on the news every night. Haiti is where people have tuberculosis. Haiti is where people eat cats. You do not represent Haiti at all to them anymore. You are an aberration because you look like them and you talk like them. They do not see you. They do not see the worlds that have made you. You want to say to them that you are Haiti, too. Your house is Haiti, too, and what does that do to their perceptions? You have the choice of passing but you don't. You claim your *dyaspora* status hoping it will force them to expand their image of what Haiti is but it doesn't. Your sister who is younger and very sensitive begins to deny that she is Haitian. She is American, she says. American.

You turn to books to lose yourself. You read stories about people from other places. You read stories about people from here. You read stories about people from other places who now live here. You decide you will become a writer. Through your writing they will see you, *dyaspora* child, the connections and disconnections that have made you the mosaic that you are. They will see where you are from and the worlds that have made you. They will see you.

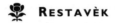

RESTAVÈK

Jean-Robert Cadet

"A *blan* (white person) is coming to visit today. He's your papa, but when you see him, don't call him papa. Say *'Bonjour, monsieur'* and disappear. If the neighbors ask who he was, you tell them that you don't know. He is such a good man, we have to protect his reputation. That's what happens when men of good character have children with dogs," said Florence to me in *Kreyòl* when I was about seven or eight years old. Before noon, a small black car pulled into the driveway and a white man got out of it. As I made eye contact with him, he waved at me and quickly stepped up to the front door before I had a chance to say *"Bonjour, monsieur."* Florence let him into the house and I disappeared into the backyard. Almost immediately I heard him leaving.

At the age of five I had begun to hate Florence. "I wish your *manman* was my *manman* too," I told Eric, a little boy my age who lived next door. One day while we played together, Eric's mother pulled a handkerchief from her bra, wet its corner on her tongue, knelt down on one knee, and wiped off a dirty spot on her son's face. Eric pushed her hand away.

"Ah, *Manman*, stop it," he said.

I looked at her with bright eyes. "Do it to me instead," I said.

She stared at my face for a moment and replied with an affectionate smile, "But your face is not dirty."

To which I answered, "I don't care. Do it to me anyway." She gently wiped at a spot on my face, as I grinned from ear to ear.

My biological mother had died before her image was ever etched in my mind. I cannot remember the time when I was brought to Florence, the woman I called *Manman*. She was a beautiful Negress with a dark-brown complexion and a majestic presence. She had no job, but earned a small income from tenants who leased her inherited farmland. She also entertained high government officials as a means to supplement her income. Her teenage son, Denis, was living with his paternal grandmother and attending private school. Florence claimed that her husband had died when her son was ten years old, but I never saw her wedding pictures.

I came into Florence's life one day when Philippe, her white former lover, paid her a surprise visit. He was a successful exporter of coffee and chocolate to the United States and Europe. Philippe lived in Port-au-Prince, Haiti, with his parents, two brothers, and a niece. He arrived in his Jeep at Florence's two-story French country-style house in an upper-class section of the city. A bright-eyed, fat-cheeked, light-skinned black baby boy was in the backseat. Philippe parked the car, reached into the back seat, and took the baby out. He stood him on the ground and the baby toddled off. I was that toddler.

Philippe greeted Florence with a kiss on each cheek while she stared at the toddler. "Whose baby is this?" she asked, knowing the answer to her question.

"His mother died and I can't take him home to my parents. I'd like you to have him," said Philippe, handing Florence an envelope containing money.

"I understand," she said, taking the envelope. He embraced her again and drove off, leaving me behind. Philippe's problem was solved.

My mother had been a worker in one of Philippe's coffee factories below the Cahos mountains of the Artibonite Valley. Like the grand *blans* of the distant past who acknowledged their blood in the veins of their slave children by emancipating and educating them, Philippe was following tradition. Perhaps he thought that Florence would give me a better life.

"Angela," yelled Florence.

"Oui, Madame," answered the cook, approaching her.

"Take care of this little boy, will you? Find him something to eat," she instructed. Angela picked me up.

"What's his name?" she asked.

Florence thought for a moment and said, "Bobby." Florence did not want another child, but the financial arrangement she had with Philippe was too attractive for her to turn down. Every night I slept on a pile of rags in a corner of Florence's bedroom, like a house cat, until I was six years old. Then she made me sleep under the kitchen table.

Florence did not take care of me. From the time I entered the household, various cooks met my basic needs, which freed Florence from having to deal with me. I was never greatly attached to any of the cooks, since none of them ever lasted for more than a year. Florence would fire them for burning a meal or for short-changing her when they returned from the market.

As I got older, I learned what kind of day I was going to have based on Florence's mood and tone of voice. When she was cheerful, the four-strip leather whip, called a *matinèt,* would stay hung on its hook against the kitchen wall.

I knew of two groups of children in Port-au-Prince: the elite, and the very poor, the *restavèks,* or slave children.

Children of the elite are often recognized by their light skin and the fine quality of their clothes. They are encouraged by their parents to speak proper French instead of *Kreyòl*, the language of the masses. They live in comfortable homes with detached servants' quarters and tropical gardens. Their weekly spending allowance far exceeds the monthly salary of their maids. They are addressed by the maids as "Monsieur" or "Mademoiselle" before their first names. They are chauffeured to the best private schools and people call them *"ti (petit) bourgeois."*

Children of the poor often have dark skin. They appear dusty and malnourished. In their one-room homes covered with rusted sheet metal there is no running water or electricity. Their meals of red beans, cornmeal, and yams are cooked under clouds of smoke spewed out by stoves made of three coconut-size stones and fueled by dry twigs and wood. They eat from calabash bowls with their fingers and drink from tin cans with sharp edges, sitting on logs while being bothered by flies. They squat in the underbrush and wipe themselves with rocks or leaves. At night, they sleep on straw mats or cardboard spread over dirty floors while bloodsucking bedbugs feast on their sweaty flesh. They walk several miles to ill-equipped public schools, where they depend on lunches of powdered milk donated by foreign countries that once depended on the slave labor of their ancestors. After school, they rush home to recite their lessons loudly in cadence before the Caribbean daylight fades away, or they walk a few miles to Champ-de-Mars, the park, and sit under street lamps to do their homework while moths zigzag above their heads.

Restavèks are slave children who belong to well-to-do families. They receive no pay and are kept out of school. Since the emancipation and independence of 1804, affluent blacks and mulattoes have reintroduced slavery by using children of the very poor as house servants. They promise poor families in faraway villages who have

too many mouths to feed a better life for their children. Once acquired, these children lose all contact with their families and, like
the slaves of the past, are sometimes given new names for the sake
of convenience. The affluent disguise their evil deed with the label
restavèk, a term that means "staying with." Other children taunt them
with the term because they are often seen in the streets running
errands barefoot and dressed in dirty rags.

Restavèks are treated worse than slaves, because they don't cost
anything and their supply seems inexhaustible. They do the jobs that
hired domestics, or *bonnes,* will not do and are made to sleep on
cardboard, whether under the kitchen table or outside on the front
porch. For any minor infraction, they are severely whipped with the
cowhide implement that is still being made exclusively for that very
purpose. And, like the African slaves of the past, they often cook
their own meals, which are composed of inferior cornmeal and a
few heads of dried herring. Girls are usually worse off because they
are sometimes used as concubines for the teenage sons of their
"owner." And if they become pregnant, they are thrown into the
streets to earn their living as prostitutes. The boys are discarded to
become shoeshine boys or itinerant gardeners.

I was a *restavèk* in the making. Raising me as such was more
convenient for Florence, because she didn't have to explain to anyone who I was or where I came from. As a *restavèk,* I could not
interact with Florence on a personal level; I could not talk to her
about my needs. I could not speak until spoken to, except to give
her messages that third parties had left with me. I also did not dare
smile or laugh in her presence, as this would have been considered
disrespectful—I was not her son but her *restavèk*.

My tin cup, aluminum plate, and spoon were kept separate from
the regular tableware. My clothes were rags and neighborhood children shouted *"restavèk"* whenever they saw me in the streets. I always

felt hurt and deeply embarrassed, because to me the word meant motherless and unwanted. When visitors came and saw me in the yard, I was always asked. *"Ti garçon* [little boy], where is your grown-up?" Had I been wearing decent clothes and shoes, the question would have been, *"Ti monsieur* [young gentleman], where is your mother or father?"

Every night in my bedding under the kitchen table, I wished that either I or Florence would never wake up again. I wanted to live in the world of dreams where I sometimes flew like a bird and swam like a fish. But in the dream world I always stopped to relieve myself against a tree, causing me to awake in a puddle of urine.

Returning to the real world was a nightmare in itself—I was always trying to avoid Florence, the woman I called *Manman.* Every day I wished Florence would die in her sleep—until I made a most frightening discovery. While cleaning the bathroom one early evening, I noticed a small canvas bag tied into a ball under the sink. Curious, I opened it and found several pieces of bloodstained rags. Suddenly my heart raced, and I became convinced that Florence was going to die. I had a strong desire to ask her where the blood came from, but I couldn't. I was allowed to speak to Florence only when she questioned me or when I had to deliver a message from a third party.

The thought of Florence dying was real in my mind. Sometimes I sobbed, asking God to take back my wish for her death. I began to watch Florence closely, staring at every exposed part of her body, trying to find the source of the blood. I spied on her through keyholes whenever she was in the bathroom or in the bedroom.

One hot and muggy afternoon, after she pinched me and pulled me by the skin of my stomach because I had forgotten to clean the kitchen floor, she gave me a small bag of laundry detergent labeled Fab, and a bottle of Clorox bleach. "Go to the bathroom and wash the rags in the bucket," she commanded with rage. I uncovered the metal bucket and saw a pile of white rags soaking in bloody water. I reached in the bucket and scrubbed each piece until the stains began to fade. I vomited in the toilet and continued with my chore.

After a small eternity, Florence opened the door. Fresh air rushed in and I filled my lungs. My ragged shirt was soaked with sweat. I looked up and realized for the first time that Florence was the tallest woman I had ever known. After she inspected the rags, she said, "Now soak them in the bleach. Tomorrow you can rinse them." As I followed her instructions, I stared at her feet, searching again for the source of the blood.

The following day, without being told, I scrubbed the rags again, one by one, and rinsed each piece. As I hung them to dry over the clothesline in the backyard, Florence came out to observe. "After they're dry, fold them and put them in this," she said as she handed me the small white canvas bag. I took it from her, scanning her arms and legs for scars. She had none.

I replied, *"Oui"* instead of the usual *"Oui, Manman."* At the end of the day, I followed her instructions and placed the bag on her bed. From then on, every month, Florence handed me the small white canvas bag with laundry detergent and commanded me to wash its contents.

Every day I lived with anxiety, wondering how soon my only guardian would die from bleeding. Since I had to wash the rags in the late evening in the bathroom, I assumed that Florence didn't want anyone to know about the bleeding. I though that it was a secret she wanted me to keep.

As I walked through a neighbor's yard one day, I noticed a small light blue cardboard box with the word *Kotex* on it in a garbage can. I walked toward the box and stopped. I wanted the box to make a toy car, with Coke bottle caps for wheels and buttons for headlights.

While no one was watching, I took the box quickly, put it under my shirt, and fled. I hid it behind a bush at the side of Florence's house, waiting for free time to make a toy. After midday dinner, Florence lay down on her bed for her afternoon nap and called me in to scratch the bottom of her feet. I once heard that this was an activity female slaves used to perform for their mistresses. I despised this routine because I had to kneel at the foot of the bed on the mosaic floor, causing my abscessed right knee to hurt and ooze a foul-smelling liquid. Whenever I fell asleep at her feet, she would kick me in the face and shout, "You're going to scratch my feet until I fall asleep if I have to kick your head off, you *extrait caca* (essence of shit), you son of a whore." As Florence slept, I quickly left the room, thinking of the Kotex box I had hidden away. Once outside I crouched down and pulled the treasured box from the bush. I noticed several rolls of cloth material inside. I unrolled the first once and discovered a big bloodstain on it. Confused, I dropped it and went back to the neighbor's yard. I watched everyone's exposed skin surreptitiously, hoping to discover the source of the blood. I returned home and disposed of the box.

I sat under the mango tree in the yard with my catechism trying to memorize as much as I could in preparation for my first communion. As I recited passages, I visualized myself wearing long white pants, a white long-sleeved shirt, red bow tie, and shiny black shoes. Entering the church with my classmates, I was at the communion rail, the priest said, "The body of Christ," and I answered, "Amen" as I opened my mouth to receive the Host. I didn't imagine a big dinner reception with a house full of friends and relatives who brought gifts and money for me, but I was certain that I was going to have my first communion because my school—École du Canada—was preparing a group of students for the sacrament. I was probably eight or ten years old at the time.

During classes on Saturday afternoons, everyone was eager to answer questions and display his knowledge of the Bible and catechism. Every class started the same way.

Teacher: What is catechism?

Students: A catechism is a little book from which we learn the Catholic religion.

Teacher: Where is God?

Students: God is in heaven, on earth, and everywhere.

Teacher: Recite the Ten Commandments of God.

Thou shalt not have other gods besides me.

Thou shalt not . . .

Thou shalt not . . .

Everyone responded to every question and command in unison and with enthusiasm. At the end of the class, we told each other with gleaming eyes what our parents planned to prepare for dinner the day of the first communion. It seemed that everyone's parents had been fattening either a goat or a turkey. Some talked about their trip to the tailor or the shoemaker. Everyone had a story to tell— even I, but my stories were all made up. During every trip back home, I thought about the First Commandment and wondered why Florence worshipped several other gods immediately after she returned home from church. She must have known about the Ten Commandments, because I read them in her prayer book every time she visited her neighbors.

Saturday evening, the week before confession, the students were very excited, knowing the day of the first communion was getting closer. After class, everyone told stories of how his shoes and clothes were delivered or picked up. At home, I searched Florence's bedroom for new clothes and shoes and found nothing that belonged to me. I wanted to ask Florence if she had purchased the necessary clothes for me, but I could not, since I wasn't allowed to ask her questions. I considered asking her anyway and taking the risk of being slapped. But I couldn't vocalize the words—my fear of her was too intimidating. Thursday afternoon, I searched again in every closet and under the bed and found nothing.

I began to worry. Maybe she forgot, I thought. I placed the catechism on the dining-room table as a reminder to Florence. She placed it on the kitchen table instead. "She remembers," I said to myself with a grin.

Friday afternoon, the evening of confession, a street vendor was heard hawking her goods. "Bobby, call the vendor," yelled Florence. I ran to the sidewalk and summoned the woman vendor, who had coal-black skin and was balancing a huge yellow basket on top of her head. Several chickens with colorful plumage were hung upside down from her left forearm. Once in the yard and under the tree, she bent down and placed the pile of poultry on the ground. Florence's cook assisted her in freeing her head from the heavy load. After several minutes of bargaining, Florence bought two chickens. I felt very happy, thinking that a big dinner was being planned to celebrate my first communion. But deep down inside, a small doubt lingered. Saturday morning, the eve of my first communion, Florence left in a taxi. I had never been so happy. "*Manman* went to buy clothes for my first communion," I told the cook, smiling, dancing, and singing. She paid no attention to me, but the expression on her face dampened my festive mood. By noon a taxi stopped in front to the house. I ran to see. It was Florence, carrying a big brown paper bag. I danced in my heart as I fought against the urge to hug her, knowing she would slap me away.

She walked in without saying a word. I went inside and fetched her slippers. She changed into another dress and began to supervise the cook, who was preparing dinner. In the early afternoon, after I finished my chores, I approached Florence with a pail of water and a towel and began to wash her feet. She was sitting in her rocking chair, sipping sweet hot black coffee from a saucer. With pounding heart, I spoke, "Confession is at six o'clock and communion is tomorrow at nine o'clock in the morning."

She stared at me for a long moment as she ground her teeth. Her face turned very angry. "You little shithead bedwetter, you little faggot, you shoeshine boy. If you think I'm gonna spend my money on your first communion, you're insane," she shouted. Trembling with fear, I dried her feet, slipped on her slippers, and stood up, holding the pail and towel. I felt as though my feet and legs were too heavy for me to move. I was stunned by her words. "Get out of my face," she yelled. I went into the kitchen and sat quietly in my usual corner without shedding a tear.

"Amelia!" called Florence loudly.

"*Oui*, Madame Cadet," the cook responded.

"You don't need to prepare the chicken for tomorrow; I'm spending the day with my niece. Her son is having his first communion tomorrow," she said.

I went to her bedroom to find out the contents of the bag and saw a pair of shoes she intended to wear to her godson's first communion. I felt crushed, but at the same time resigned myself to believe that only children with real mothers and fathers go to communion, receive presents from Santa Claus, and celebrate their birthdays.

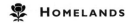 **HOMELANDS**

Marie-Hélène Laforest

My truth, like many truths, is partial. As I set out to tell this story, I suspect the other characters involved would tell it differently. Only on one point would my relatives and I agree: we had not been black before leaving the Caribbean. In a country of dark-skinned people, my lighter skin color and my family's wealth made me white. My white grandfather was a coffee and sisal exporter in a small town to the north of Port-au-Prince. He conducted his business out of his general store, which imported construction materials and basic food-stuffs like flour. He was the honorary consul of Norway. Before the National Bank of Haiti closed for the weekend on Fridays, a large trunk painted green, full of his money, was put onto a dray, held in place with a thick rope, and pushed by a bare-chested man through the Grande Rue to the bank. My grandfather's half-brother had brown skin and green eyes. Perhaps my grandfather had a better knack for business, but I could not help thinking, as a child, that his skin color put him on the Grande Rue whereas his half-brother conducted his business on a back street near the market. My grand-mother's brother, too, had his business on the main street. He was light-skinned and his wife was a woman whose veins showed through her white skin. The Europeans, mostly the clergy, and the

Canadians, who exploited a copper mine in the area, patronized my grandfather's and his brother-in-law's businesses.

I had not been a "Caribbean" either before leaving Haiti. I knew a few of the other islands by name but had not met anyone from there. My mother and her sister had gone to Cuba for their trousseaus. They spoke of Havana City being like Paris, but they spoke of it in the past tense. It had lost its glamour after Fidel Castro took over. When I was six years old, my mother took me on a trip to Miami to see the Seminoles on their reservation and the dolphins in the Seaquarium. There was a stopover in Montego Bay, Jamaica. I was allowed to stand by the plane door before the Jamaican passengers boarded. Rows and rows of people stood away from the tarmac behind a wire fence, none black, all Chinese. I ran inside to inform my mother we had landed in China. Little did I know that thirty years after this incident I would be taken for a Caribbean person of Chinese ancestry by a group of Jamaicans.

On the island of my birth, my life of privilege was constructed with great conviction. There were many invisible lines marking off paths from which I could not swerve. I remember one October, on the first day of school, dressed in my starched blue uniform, waiting for my father and the oyster man. A huge mango gropo tree grew in our backyard by the pool side, a green-and-white-leaf vine coiled around its trunk. My father sat underneath that tree to have his shoes cleaned by the shoeshine man at his feet. At the same time, the oyster man arrived and cracked open the oysters, which we slurped down with a dash of lemon. My father drove to work. The yardman took me to school on his bicycle. Sometimes we took the hospital road where we passed men carrying sick children on their backs in the bright morning sun. This is the image the word *poverty* evokes in my mind, a father traveling on foot to a faraway hospital, his sick child on his back.

Walking back from school, I stopped first at my great uncle's store, where he and his wife interrupted their activities to hug and kiss me and give me presents in the form of candies or, if I had received my report card that day, perfumes, jewelry, or pieces of fabric from England or France. Broderie anglaise was my favorite. Then I proceeded to my grandfather's shop. At lunchtime, my grandfather drove me to the two-story house with the balcony skirting the top floor where my grandmother sat on her rocking chair. Lunch was always our favorite food. My grandfather and I both liked food that was considered too ordinary for people with means: *tchaka*, *akra*, crabs, fish stew and cornmeal, salted fish and boiled bananas. After lunch, while my grandparents napped, I went down to the ground floor. The back door opened onto the yard where the numerous household workers lived: the cook, the two housemaids with their children, the woman who ironed, the boy who cleaned the yard, the boy who did errands. This was another world, a life of chatter, of blue indigo, thick white corn starch, scallions, hot peppers, coffee beans roasting on a wood fire, a world where many things were done at once. The women hulled peas, ironed clothes, sang, plaited hair, reprimanded the children, and laughed. For me it was the place where I could eat with a spoon instead of a fork, even with my hands, a place where I spoke *Kreyòl* instead of French and learned riddles and songs. I preferred staying there to spending time upstairs or at my parents' house, where I had no playmates.

My parents' house stood away from the center of town. Our property was surrounded by almond, mango, and palm trees, a barrier before the vast extension of sugarcane fields. Our closest neighbors were the poor farmers of the area. This was my brothers' realm. My brothers played with the boys their age, climbing trees, carving bows from branches, chasing birds with slingshots, making kites. As a girl I was seldom allowed to play with them. My only playmate and friend was Yanyan, a young *restavèk* girl who lived at my grandmother's house. She was older than me, old enough to be in charge of me and my cousins when they visited, but young enough to play with us. She came on car rides, Sunday outings to the river; we jumped rope and picked mangoes from trees together. Yanyan and I were always together except when I was called for lunch or dinner. I went upstairs, she stayed downstairs in the yard in the maids' quarters. Church was yet another moment of social separation for Yanyan and me. She went to the four o'clock Sunday Mass, the one the priests said at the cathedral for house servants who started their day's work at six in the morning, grinding or brewing coffee to be brought to their employers' bedside by seven. I went to ten o'clock Mass and sat in the front-row pew, paid for by my family and reserved for us. Yanyan's brother and mother visited my grandmother's yard, most often to eat. If my parents were not there, my grandmother would give me permission to join Yanyan and the maids and their families in the evening. If my parents were present, I had to tiptoe my way down the wooden stairs to the back of the house where everyone sat on low chairs and told riddles and stories. The cook was the best narrator. Her stories were all interspersed with songs. All the tales ended with "someone kicked me and that's how I got here to tell you this story." With me, Yanyan spoke a mixture of *Kreyòl* and French, with the adults, she only spoke *Kreyòl*, fearing their scorn. At the dinner table in my family no one was allowed to speak *Kreyòl* and no child could address an adult in the family in *Kreyòl*. Our command of French reaffirmed our social status.

One day in March 1963 my father, a factory owner, had to leave the island. A few weeks earlier, he had been arrested by François Duvalier's henchmen while we were attending Sunday Mass. My father and his friends would usually stand in the back of the church and step out right after communion. Before the priest pronounced *"Ite Missa*

est," they would already be chatting on the church steps. We noticed
my father's absence when the service was over. It was not clear to me
why he was arrested. Was it because he had attended the military academy in his youth? The other four taken to the police station that day
were men who were loved by everyone, men who'd had no connections to the military. What my father and those men all had in common was that they were light-skinned Haitians, members of the
so-called "elite." The next morning all five were freed. Their arrest
was a rehearsal for what would follow—Duvalier's reign of terror.

A few weeks after my father's brief detention, he closed his factory
in Port-au-Prince and left for New York. My mother, my brothers
and sister, and I were to join him there at the end of the school year.
In the months in which we were separated, many of our neighbors'
houses were burned down and schools often stayed closed. At the
end of June our exile began.

New York held no welcome signs for us. We lived in one of the
many peripheral cities within the City, in a world made of Cuban
and South American exiles, surrounded by white Americans. We
moved into a building in Elmhurst, Queens, where two Haitian
families, the very first victims of Duvalier's purge, had settled. They
had taken refuge in foreign embassies and then found their way to
New York. One of them was my mother's cousin. Through him
we were able to rent an apartment in an attractive eight-story building with two elevators. Unlike the wide-open spaces we had left on
the island where kites had risen into the infinite sky, the apartment
building called for hushed voices and quietness. We did not speak
in the hallways or in the elevator. When we encountered our white
American neighbors, they could not help but stare at us. Their silence
was ominous like their stares. I did not associate this with racism
until much later. Our very presence, it seemed, disturbed the world
they had created for themselves. To them we had no right to these

surroundings, to settle on their street. From one day to the next they were all gone, as if they had boarded the same ship. The clean-shaven superintendent—thanks to whom the fountain surrounded with ferns in the lobby hissed all day—left in their wake. The new super wore dirty, sleeveless undershirts and spoke unintelligible English. He did not clean the lobby; the fountain stopped spouting water.

While my brothers, sister, and I were forced to gain quick familiarity with things American, our parents remained suspended between New York and Haiti, the past and the present. Puzzled by events such as semiformals and proms, inviting boys to dance, and wearing corsages on wrists, I received no help at home. I remember writing notes to my teachers and my brothers' teachers for my mother to sign. I became her substitute, speaking to the teachers, buying my younger siblings school uniforms. In the daytime the male adults in our little group were dispersed throughout the city, each busy with his own survival. They traveled huge distances in subway cars while the women, still refusing to eat off of paper plates or bring food home in Styrofoam containers, wept for the loss of home. My mother became a housewife, which meant doing the work the numerous household help had done for her in Haiti. There was very little talking within our apartment walls, as if each one of us was pondering alone on his or her lot in the new spaces we'd come to inhabit. Communication with home was costly and difficult. No direct phone lines to Haiti. No traveling back and forth. We lived with the desire to return.

Six years into our exile, our former house help, who had since migrated, came to visit us. Their fur stoles and fashionable hairstyles indicated that they were making a nice living for themselves. Unlike those of us who were waiting for the Duvalier reign to end in order to go home, they had no intention of returning, no desire to give up

material well-being and the advance in social status that they had acquired here. We hugged them, exchanged a few pleasantries, talked
about their families and ours, about former neighbors. I wondered
about Yanyan. I'd heard that she had gotten pregnant and was living
with her mother in a shack not far from the wharf in our hometown.
She was among the ones who would never make it to New York.

When our visitors left, my family considered the oddness of it all,
the apparent leveling that American society offered, seeing us all as
equally black.

There was a club in Port-au-Prince—it probably still exists today—
in which the members' skin tone went from white to brown to dark
brown. Those of pure African ancestry and those who could not
afford the high yearly fees could not belong. It was a place in which
people did not need to be introduced to each other, where people
were known by their family names. While the children would sit by
the pool and order sandwiches, Cokes, and ice cream, their parents
would play bridge or tennis. The club's name was Bellevue. My
cousins and I spent many Saturday afternoons by the Bellevue pool,
which was larger and had a higher diving board than the ones we
had in our homes. There and elsewhere children like me were
trained to accept our privileged status, to see ourselves as separate
from the rest of the population, as if we came from a superior breed.
There and elsewhere we learned the nuances in glances which indicate degrees of familiarity or lack of acknowledgment.

I was never aware of the fact that I don't look at people who are
considered social inferiors to me in the eyes, until my Italian husband
recently pointed it out to me in our home in Naples. It was then
that I realized that whiteness was rarely mentioned in my family,
blackness often. Dark-skinned people who frequented our homes
were hand-picked: my grandfather's best friend whom he saw every

day; my mother's school friend and my grandmother's old neighbor who came and went as they pleased. There were others, too, but they had been singled out. In our family, wholesale acceptance of blackness was unthinkable. My mother had an obsession with her lower lip and consequently with mine, reminding me all the time to pull it in, something I found impossible to do. When my hair was loose she called it a *papousserie*, a French term deriving from their descriptions of the people of Papua.

One day in July 1969—I had taken a summer job in a department store on Queens Boulevard—an African-American girl asked me if any "brothers" had been hired. Brothers? I wondered. I did not know what she meant. It was one of the most embarrassing moments of my life. A revolution had started in the American world of which I was not yet aware. The black nation had been re-founded and I was part of it. African America was taking me into its fold and I willingly let it embrace me.

My new family would include all peoples of African heritage. Exile had made me black. Still, I cannot deny the influence of my later migrations, first to Puerto Rico, then to Italy. I cannot disown my grandmother's French songs and the French classics—Corneille, Racine—which some family members recited by rote. I cannot ignore the influence of my current life in Italy, my Italian husband, my Italian son. I speak five languages, I can guess meanings in several others I have not studied. As I did in my childhood between my grandmother's family room and her backyard, I straddle many borders, physical and otherwise. In recent years I have been to Grenada, Antigua, Puerto Rico, and Santo Domingo, coming always closer to the island of my birth, but never actually going back to it, never making the final journey, the dream of our years of exile. Between languages and borders, identities and colors, however, I have grieved for this. I am still grieving for it.

🌸 BONNE ANNÉE

Jean-Pierre Benoît

It is the 1960s, a cold New Year's day in New York. The men are huddled but it is not for warmth; if anything, the Queens apartment is overheated. Important matters are to be discussed. The women are off to the side, where they will not interfere. The location of the children is unimportant; they are ignored. I am in the last category, ignored but overhearing. French, English, and *Kreyòl* commingle. French, I understand. My English is indistinguishable from that of an American child. *Kreyòl*, the language of my birthplace, is a mystery. *Kreyòl* predominates, but enough is said in French and English for me to follow. He is leaving. Any day. Father Doctor. Papa Doc. Apparently he is the reason we are in New York, not Port-au-Prince. And now he is leaving. And this will make all the difference. My father is clear. We are returning to Haiti. As soon as this man leaves. No need to await the end of the school year, although my schooling is otherwise so important.

I have no memory of Haiti. No memory of my crib in Port-au-Prince, no memory of the neighbors' children or the house in which we lived. My friends are in New York. My teachers are in New York. The Mets are in New York. I do not know Papa Doc, but our destinies are linked. If he leaves, I leave. I do not want him to leave.

Another January first, another gathering. If it is the beginning of a new year, that is at best incidental. January first is the celebration of Haitian independence. A glorious day in world history, even if someone seems to have forgotten to tell the rest of the world. But it is not bygone glory that is of the moment. A new independence is dawning. It is more than just a rumor this time. Someone has inside information. It is a matter of months, weeks, maybe days, before Duvalier falls. I am one year older now, and I understand who Duvalier is. An evil man. A thief and a murderer. A monster who holds a nation prisoner. A man who tried to have my father killed. A man who will soon get his justice. My father is adamant, Duvalier's days are numbered. And then we will return. Do I want to leave? I am old enough to realize that the question is unimportant.

Go he must, but somehow he persists. A new year and he is still in power. But not for long. This time it is true. The signs are unmistakable, the gods have finally awoken. Or have they? After so many years, the debates intensify. Voices raised in excitement, in agitation, in Haitian cadences. Inevitably, hope triumphs over history. Or ancient history triumphs over recent history. Perhaps there will be a coup, Haitian exiles landing on the shores with plans and weapons, a well-timed assassination.

We are not meant to be in this country. We did not want to come. We were forced to flee or die. Americans perceive desperate brown masses swarming at their golden shores, wildly inventing claims of persecution for the opportunity to flourish in this prosperous land. The view from beneath the bridge is somewhat different: reluctant refugees with an aching love of their forsaken homeland, of a homeland that has forsaken them, refugees who desire nothing more than to be home again.

Then there are the children. Despite having been raised in the United States, I have no special love for this country. Despite the searing example of my elders, I am not even sure what it means to love a country. Clearly, it is not the government that one is to love. Is it then the land, the dirt and the grass, the rocks and the hills? The people? Are one people any better than another? I have no special love for this country, but neither do I desire a return to a birthplace that will, in fact, be no real return at all. If nothing else, the United States is the country that I know, English is my daily language. Another New Year, but I am not worried; we will not be back in Port-au-Prince anytime soon. With their crooked ruler the adults can no longer draw a straight line, but I can still connect the dots and see that they lead nowhere.

I I

The Haitian sun has made the cross-Atlantic journey to shine on her dispossessed children. This time it is not just wispy speculation, something has changed. It is spring 1971 and there is death to celebrate. The revolutionaries have not landed on the coast, the assassin's poison has not found its blood. Nonetheless, Duvalier is dead. Unnaturally, he has died of natural causes. Only his laughable son remains. *Bébé* Doc, Jean-Claude Duvalier. Everyone agrees that *Bébé* Doc will not be in power long enough to have his diapers changed.

Laughable *Bébé* Doc may be, but it turns out to be a long joke, and a cruel one. The father lasted fourteen years, the son will last fifteen. Twenty-nine years is a brief time in the life of a country, but a long time in the life of its people. Twenty-nine years is a very long time in the life of an exile waiting to go home.

Three years into *Bébé* Doc's terrible reign there is news of a

different sort. For the first time, Haiti has qualified for the World
Cup. The inaugural game is against eternal powerhouse Italy. In
1974 there are not yet any soccer moms, there is no ESPN all-sports
network. Americans do not know anything of soccer, and this World
Cup match will not be televised. Yet America remains a land of
immigrants. For an admission fee, the game will be shown at Madison Square Garden on four huge screens suspended in a boxlike
arrangement high above the basketball floor. I go with my younger
brother. In goal, Italy has the legendary Dino Zoff. Together they
have not been scored upon in two years. The poor Haitians have no
hope. And yet, Haitians hope even when there is no hope. The tri-
syllable cry of "HA-I-TI" fills the air. It meets a response, "I-TA-
LIA," twice as loud but destined to be replaced by an even louder
HA-I-TI, followed by IT-A-LIA and again HA-I-TI in a spiraling
crescendo. The game has not even started.

My brother and I join in the cheer; every time Haiti touches the
ball is cause for excitement. The first half ends scoreless. The Italian
fans are nervous, but the Haitian fans are feeling buoyed. After all,
Haiti could hardly be expected to score a goal, not when the Ger-
mans and the English and the Brazilians before them have failed to
penetrate the Italian defense. At the same time, the unheralded Haitian defenders have held. The second half begins. Less than a minute
has gone by and Emanuel Sanon, the left-winger for Haiti, has the
ball. Less than twenty-four hours earlier he had foolhardily predicted
that he will score. Zoff is fully aware of him. Sanon shoots. There
is a split second of silence and then madness. The ball is in the back
of the net, Sanon has beaten Zoff. The Italians are in shock. The
world is in shock. Haiti leads 1–0.

"HA-I-TI, HA-I-TI." Half of Madison Square Garden is deliri-
ous, half is uncomprehending. The Haitians are beating the Italians.
Haiti is winning. Haiti is winning. For six minutes. Then the Italians

come back to tie the score, 1–1. The Italians score again. And then again. The Haitians cannot respond. Italy wins 3–1.

Still. Still, for six minutes Haiti is doing the impossible, Haiti is beating Italy. Italy, which twice has won the World Cup. Six minutes. Perhaps the natal pull is stronger than it seems. For that one goal, that brief lead, those six minutes, mean more to me than all the victories of my favorite baseball team.

III

February 7, 1986, amid massive protests in Haiti, Jean-Claude flees the country. There is a blizzard in New York, but this does not prevent jubilant Haitians from taking to the snowy streets, waving flags, honking horns, pouring champagne. Restaurants in Brooklyn serve up free food and drink. The Duvalier regime has finally come to an end. The New Year's prediction has finally come true. If he leaves, I leave. In July, I fulfill my destiny, more or less. I return to Haiti, on an American passport, for a two-week visit.

In October the Mets win their second World Series. The city celebrates with a tickertape parade attended by over two million people. A pale celebration indeed, compared to the celebrating that took place earlier in the year.

🌹 HAITI: A MEMORY JOURNEY

Assotto Saint

Early Friday morning, February 7, 1986, drinking champagne and watching televised reports of Haitian President-for-Life Jean-Claude "Baby Doc" Duvalier fleeing for his life aboard a U.S. Air Force plane, I can't help but reminisce about my childhood experiences, and reflect on the current political and social situation, along with my expectations as a gay man who was born and grew up there.

Having seen, so many times during the AIDS crisis, Haitian doctors and community leaders deny the existence of homosexuality in Haiti; having heard constantly that the first afflicted male cases in Haiti were not homosexual, but alas, poor hustlers who were *used* by visiting homosexual American tourists who infected them and thus introduced the disease into the country; having felt outrage at the many excuses, lies, denials, and apologies—I am duty-bound to come out and speak up for the thousands of Haitians like me, gay and not hustlers, who for one reason or another, struggle with silence and anonymity yet don't view themselves as victims. Self-pity simply isn't part of my vocabulary. Haunted by the future, I'm desperate to bear witness and settle accounts. These are trying times. These are times of need.

For years now, Haiti has not been a home but a cause to me.

Many of my passions are still there. Although I did my best to distance myself from the homophobic Haitian community in New York, to bury painful emotions in my accumulated memories of childhood, I was politically concerned and committed to the fight for change in my native land. It's not surprising that the three hardest yet most exhilarating decisions I have faced had to do with balancing my Haitian roots and gay lifestyle. The first was leaving Haiti to live in the United States. The second was going back to meet my father for the first time. The third, tearing up my application to become a U.S. citizen. Anytime one tries to take fragments of one's personal mythology and make them understandable to the whole world, one reaches back to the past. It must be dreamed again.

I was born on October 2, 1957, one week after François (Papa Doc) Duvalier was elected president. He had been a brilliant doctor and a writer of great verve from the *Griots* (negritude) movement. Until that time, the accepted images of beauty in Haiti, the images of "civilization," tended to be European. Fair skin and straight hair were better than dark and kinky. Duvalier was black pride. Unlike previous dictators who had ruled the country continuously since its independence from the French in 1804, Duvalier was not mulatto, and he did not surround himself with mulattoes, a mixed-race group that controlled the economy. Duvalier brought *Vodou* to the forefront of our culture and, later in his reign, used it to tyrannize the people.

I grew up in Les Cayes, a sleepy port city of twenty thousand in southwest Haiti, where nothing much happened. Straight A's, ran like a girl, cute powdered face, silky eyebrows—I was the kind of child folks saw and thought quick something didn't click. I knew very early on that I was "different," and I was often reminded of that fact by my schoolmates. *"Masisi"* (faggot), they'd tease me. That word to this day sends shivers down my spine but, being the town's best-behaved child, a smile, a kind word were my winning numbers.

We—my mother (a registered nurse anesthetist), grandfather (a lawyer who held, at one time or another, each of the town's top official posts, from mayor on down), grandmother, and I—lived in a big beautiful house facing the cathedral. The Catholic Mass, especially High Mass on Sundays and holy days, with its colorful pageantry, trance-inducing liturgy, and theatrical ceremony, spellbound me. And that incense—that incense took me heaven-high each time. I was addicted and I attended Mass every day. Besides, I had other reasons. I had developed a mad crush on the parish priest, a handsome Belgian who sang like a bird.

I must have been seven when I realized my attraction to men. Right before first communion, confused and not making sense, I confessed to this priest. Whether he understood me or not, he gave me absolution and told me to say a dozen Hail Marys. Oh Lord, did I pray. Still girls did nothing for me. Most of my classmates had girlfriends to whom they sent passionate love poems and sugar candies, and whom they took to movies on Sunday afternoons. All I wanted to do with girls was skip rope, put makeup on their faces, and comb their hair. I was peculiar.

Knowing that I probably would never marry, I decided that I wanted to be a priest when I grew up. For one, priests are celibate, and I had noticed that they were effeminate. Some even lisped, like me. I built a little altar in my bedroom with some saints' icons, plastic lilies, and colored candles and dressed in my mother's nursing uniform and petticoat. I said Mass every night. The archbishop of Haiti, François W. Ligondé, a childhood friend of my mother and uncles, even blessed my little church when he once visited my family. I was so proud. Everybody felt that I'd be the perfect priest, except my mother, who I later found out wanted me to become a doctor like my father—who I never met, never saw pictures of, never heard mention of, and accepted as a nonentity in my life.

I used to believe that I was born by immaculate conception, until one day I was ridiculed in school by my science teacher, who had asked me for my father's name. When I told him of my belief, he laughed and got the entire class to laugh along. Until then I had never questioned the fact that my last name was the same as that of my mother, who was not married. It was then that I smelled foul play and suspected that I was the result of sexual relations between my mother and grandfather. I didn't dare ask.

In the early 1960s, Papa Doc declared himself President-for-Life and things got worse and worse. I remember hearing of anti-Duvalier suspects being arrested. I remember hearing of families being rounded up and even babies being killed. I remember the mysterious disappearances at night, the mutilated corpses being found by roads and rivers the next day. I remember the public slayings, adults whispering and sending my cousins and me to another room so they could talk. Rumors of invasions by exiled Haitians abounded. Some of these invasions were quickly stopped by government forces. The *tonton macoutes* (bogeymen) were everywhere, with their rifles slung over their shoulders and their eyes of madness and cruelty.

Poverty was all around me and, in my child-mind, I had accepted this. Some had, some had not. Fate. Cyclones, hurricanes, floods came and went. Carnival was always a happy time, though. Dressed in a costume, I, along with thousands, took to the streets each year with our favorite music bands. Grandmother died during Mardi Gras '65. I was miserable for weeks and kept a daily journal to her. Soon after, mother left for Switzerland and I moved in with my aunt Marcelle and her husband.

In 1968, my aunt had her first and only child. Was I jealous! I had been quite comfortable and so spoiled for three years that when she gave birth to Alin, it was difficult for me to accept that I was not her real child, a fact I had, at times, forgotten. That year she gave me a beautiful birthday party. My schoolmates were making fun of me more than ever. I still wanted to be a priest. I said a Mass for Martin Luther King, Jr., and Bobby Kennedy when each was assassinated. Duvalier declared himself the flag of the nation and became more ruthless. I took long walks on the beach by myself. It was a year of discovery.

One afternoon, I saw Pierre swimming alone. He called me to join him. I was surprised. Although we went to the same school and we had spoken to each other once or twice, we were not buddies. Three or four years older, tall and muscular, Pierre was a member of the volleyball team and must have had two or three girlfriends. I didn't have a swimsuit, so I swam naked. I remember the uneasiness each time our eyes met, the tension between us, my hard-on. We kept smelling each other out. He grabbed me by the waist. I felt his dick pressing against my belly. Taut smiles. I held it in my hand and it quivered. I had never touched another boy's dick before. I asked him if he had done this with other boys. He said only with girls. Waves.

He turned me around and pushed his dick in my ass. Shock. I remember the pain. Hours later, the elation I felt, knowing that another person who was like me existed. In Les Cayes, there had been rumors about three or four men who supposedly were homosexual, but they were all married. Some had no fewer than seven children. Knowing Pierre was a turning point for me. The loneliness of thinking that I was the only one with homosexual tendencies subsided.

In 1969, man walked on the moon. I was happy. Pierre and I met each other three or four times (once in my grandfather's study, and he almost caught us). I didn't say anything about this to anyone, not even at confession. I didn't pray as much. I passed my *certificat*, which is like graduation from junior high school in the U.S. Mother moved from Geneva to New York City, where I visited her in the summer of 1970. To me, New York was the Empire State Building, the Statue of Liberty, hot dogs and hamburgers, white people everywhere, museums, rock music, twenty-four-hour television, stores, stores, and subways.

I remember the day I decided to stay in the U.S. A week before I was to go back to Haiti, my mother and I were taking a trip to Coney Island. Two effeminate guys in outrageous short shorts and high heels walked onto the train and sat in front of us. Noticing that I kept looking at them, my mother said to me that this was the way it was here. People could say and do whatever they wanted; a few weeks earlier thousands of homosexuals had marched for their rights.

Thousands! I was stunned. I kept thinking what it would be like to meet some of them. I kept fantasizing that there was a homosexual world out there I knew nothing of. I remember looking up in amazement as we walked beneath the elevated train, then telling mother I didn't want to go back to Haiti. She warned me of snow, muggers, homesickness, racism, alien cards, and that I would have to learn to speak English. She warned me that our lives wouldn't be a vacation. She would have to go back to work as a night nurse in a week, and I'd have to assume many responsibilities. After all, she was a single mother.

That week, I asked her about my father and found out that they had been engaged for four years while she was in nursing school and he in medical school. She got pregnant and he wanted her to abort. A baby would have been a burden so early in their careers, especially since they planned to move to New York after they got married. Mother wouldn't abort. She couldn't. Though the two families tried to avoid a scandal and patch things up, accusations were made, and feelings hurt. Each one's decision final, they became enemies for life.

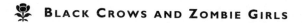

BLACK CROWS AND ZOMBIE GIRLS

Barbara Sanon

Gendarme Janeau, the officer at the Casernes de Jeremie—the local military jail house—had been summoned by the neighbors to come save our house from evil. All was quiet, for his two prisoners had been fed their daily dose of cornmeal and beans, so Janeau ran, baton and rifle in hand, to our gate. And there it was, a large black crow circling over our roof. I held on tightly to my mother's skirt to see if it would shield me until some miracle put an end to the bird's targeted prowling. Unable to find another solution, Gendarme Janeau fired into the air. The sound lingered for minutes while I hid myself behind my mother as she screamed.

The black crow bled to death in front of the large oak tree where I often played with my sisters. Gendarme Janeau, still wallowing in his triumph, convinced my mother that the crow was indeed a lustful evil spirit.

"Keep a watch out for it," he told my mother. "If it is restless, it might return. It does not get enough pleasure at night so it comes in the heat when the sun shines brightest to continue its seduction."

My mother, alone in a house with five children and a husband in New York, trembled as she took my hand and led me inside the house. For years, the townspeople would recount the tale of the

black bird and Gendarme Janeau's ability to shoot anything that
looked him in the eye too directly.

Janeau became the town hero and secretly my terror. That night,
I dreamt of the *gendarme* again killing the black crow. I dreamt of
his large hands around the black crow's neck as it screeched. In the
dream, I draped my mother's skirt to cover the bird's blood on the
ground, but the blood seeped through the cloth and Janeau, watching, smirked, amused by my naiveté.

The next day, I cringed as I rushed past the Casernes on my way
to school, fearing that I would have to stand still, frozen in place,
during the Casernes' 8:30 a.m. salute when Gendarme Janeau raised
the black-and-red Duvalierist flag that he would kill for.

Every night after that, I saw the shadow of Janeau's hand moving
above my head. Somewhere, through the window in the distance,
a light would flicker on and off and I would think that it was him
reminding me that even in my house, in my own bed, I could not
escape him. He became the bogeyman and I was his prisoner. My
sister would tell me to close my eyes under the covers in order to
prevent him from seeing me.

"Let the bad spirits pass by on their way and not look at us," she
would say. "For any contact with them will make us their victims
forever." My mother could not help us for she, too, was afraid. So
we lay quietly in the dark, waiting for the evil to pass.

A few years later, in my mother's bedroom in New York, I would
see the bogeyman again. Like the lustful crow, he, too, appeared in
the daytime in the form of my mother's boyfriend—the man who
was supposed to replace my father. This man, my mother's boyfriend, wrapped his familiar arms around my frail ten-year-old body,
drawing me with his warm smile toward his lap. How paternal he
seemed, pretending that he was offering me a warm place to sit—a
warm place to be a child. In that moment, as he fondled my body,

I decided that I was dead. My body was as ice cold as all the dead relatives' foreheads we children were made to kiss at family wakes. *I* heard voices but they could not hear *me*, for I was choking on the dirt my mother's boyfriend threw on my corpse as his nails kept on digging, digging—restless—until he reached my skeleton.

I was dead but no one realized it. People were too busy reviving the favorite Haitian pastime called political discussion. The ousting of Duvalier and the stories surrounding the event inevitably found their way into all community functions, baptisms, communions, weddings, and funerals.

Maybe one day, I thought, there would be stories also told about me, the girl who was attacked by the bogeyman in her own mother's bedroom in broad daylight. There was no room for my own horrors in the midst of the political tales though. Mine was a story that could only be told through silences too horrific to disturb.

When family and friends assembled for gatherings, there was always a little girl there that I would recognize, a girl who would have her head down, her eyes lowered a certain way. I could always experience with her the pain of her bruised genitals hidden under immaculate petticoats that pressed her into her girlhood and kept her there so she would shut up. She was always so quiet, that girl, so confused, so *egare*, that people would joke that she was a zombie. A zombie, who in the midst of the endless political discussions on right and wrong was not allowed to disclose the bad things she swallowed.

In the mythical world, a zombie is someone who is buried alive while comatose and is then revived to serve others in whatever way they want, without questioning. A zombie is someone who has lost her soul, her will, her good angel, someone who can only regain her true self once she's been given a taste of salt. But outside this mythical world, zombies howled for their salt. Whether it was the political prisoners, the protagonists of all the political fables recounted, or the little girls whose secrets I knew too well, all these zombies were howling for their life back. Some of the political prisoners were finally beginning to be heard because of the pressure from a tenacious mass. The little girls I knew, however, were dumped deeper in their coffins by adults who were supposed to have been safeguarding them.

For the girl down the street, whose school principal demanded that she be taken away from her home for a reason none of us wanted to talk about, there was no salt. The principal said she was raped by her stepfather. But there was no mythical element to that story, nothing like the black crow spirit who had come to our house.

At least with Duvalier, we could pinpoint his kind of evil, for he smirked at the howling of the corpses under his feet. But this raped girl? Why did she need to be conquered? Why was she made a zombie? And the other girl I knew, who actually had a child by her uncle, why her? Why even talk about them, these zombie girls? Their tales were not mythical enough. Their zombification was harder to explain.

And me, without even a clear narrative, without a scar as obvious as those of the other girls, or of the political victims who could point to their burnt flesh or bullet wounds, what to make of my story? A man who had vowed to my mother and our family that he would protect us from the abandonment of my natural father, chose instead to impose his need for power on me. So, I became possessed by my fright and my shame. I had become the zombie at the dinner table, at the baptisms, the wedding receptions, the funerals. I had become the girl who sat quietly with her head lowered, her eyes on the ground, and her silence intact.

I was not alone though. We had a collective, we zombies. We began to know each other. At parties, in school, in our nightmares, we dreamt of saving each other. In some cases, this zombie state was even inherited. We were children of zombie women, a matriarchal line of silence. Whether it was 1957 or 1987, our situation had not changed. Our zombie dance began with a first outing, our first lace dress for church, our first communion, our first dance. It started with the immaculate way the white talcum powder around a girl's neck suppressed the heat and ended with a dress torn and soiled with a patch of blood. It ended with our mothers chanting softly, hoping a kinder, less lustful spirit would save us both. It ended with our mothers' careful sewing of undergarments and secretly scrubbing blood off panties long before we ever reached puberty. It ended with our mothers washing, bleaching, even boiling our panties in order to make their husbands, their cousins, their lovers, their town judges, their military officers, seem clean.

Did the zombie mothers fight? Indeed they did. They wrapped their hands around their bodies, and tightened their stomachs with layers of cloth in order to press the pain inside. They stuck wire hangers inside their young daughters and scraped the evil out. They fought with their heads lowered, their eyes fixed on the ground, using as weapons plaited hair, bright satin ribbons, dresses layered in taffeta and lace.

Our nightmares became our zombie calls. We told ourselves tales of little girls who were taken by evil spirits and never seen again until they returned as skeletons, walking, tiptoeing, dancing with their families' lies. "*Aba* Duvalier!" they shouted even as the cries of so many little girls went unheard at night.

Now I know why I dreamt of covering the dead crow with my mother's dress after it died. Now I know why even my mother's large beautiful skirt could not contain the blood. Now I know why Gendarme Janeau could smirk and force me to hide. He knew then what I didn't know. There was no place to hide.

So now in my dreams, the dead crow killed by Gendarme Janeau resurrects itself over and over again as all spirits do. Roaming endlessly, it will not die, but will try to settle near yet another black oak, seeking peace.

🌹 MIGRATION

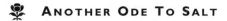 **ANOTHER ODE TO SALT**

Danielle Legros Georges

We navigate snow not ours
but grown used to, one cold foot
over another, adopt accoutrements:
a red scarf, wind-wrapped and tight,
boots, their soles teethed like sharks,
shackling our ebon ankles, the weight
of wool coats borrowed
from *our ancestors, the Gauls.*★

Masters at this now,
we circumvent ice
as we do time, reach home.

The salt you bend to cast
parts the snow around us.
I bend and think
of a primary sea,
harbors of danger and history,
passing through the middle
in boats a-sail in furious storms,

51

cargo heavy,
of *mystères,* renamed,
submerged and sure,
riding dark waves,
floating long waves
to the other side of the water,
and the other side
and the next.

★Our ancestors, the Gauls (nos ancêtres, les Gaulois)—a phrase from a French children's history text used widely, until recently, in Francophone primary schools.

🌹 AMERICA, WE ARE HERE

Dany Laferrière

I was trying to write a book and survive in America at the same time. (I'll never figure out how that ambition wormed its way into me.) One of those two pursuits had to go. Time to choose, man. But a problem arose: I wanted everything. That's the way drowning men are. I wanted a novel, girls (fascinating girls, the products of modernity, weight-loss diets, the mad longings of older men), alcohol, and laughter. My due—that's all. That's what America had promised me. I know America has made a lot of promises to a large number of people, but I was intent on making her keep her word. I was furious at her, and I don't like to be double-crossed. At the time, I'm sure you'll remember, at the beginning of the 1980s (so long ago!), the bars in any North American city were chock-full of confused, aging hippies—empty-eyed Africans who always had a drum within easy striking distance—the type never changes, no matter the location or the decade—Caribbeans in search of their identity, starving white poetesses who lived off alfalfa sprouts and Hindu mythology, aggressive young black girls who knew they didn't stand a chance in this insane game of roulette because the black men were only into white women, and the white guys into money and power. Late in the evening, I wandered through these lunar landscapes where sensations had long since replaced sentiment. I took notes. I scribbled away in the washrooms of crummy bars. I carried on endless conversations until dawn with starving intellectuals, out-of-work actresses, philosophers without influence, tubercular poetesses, the bottomest of the bottom dogs. I jumped into that pool once in a while and found myself in a strange bed with a girl I didn't remember having courted (I left the bar last night with the black-haired girl, I'm sure I did, so what's this bottle-blonde with the green fingernails doing here?) But I never took drugs. God had given me the gift of loud, powerful, happy contagious laughter, a child's laugh that drove girls wild. They wanted to laugh so badly, and there wasn't much to laugh about back then. When I immigrated to North America, I made sure I brought that laughter in my battered metal suitcase, an ancestral legacy. We always laughed a lot around my house. My grandfather's deep laughter would shake the walls. I laughed, I drank wine, I made love with the energy of a child who's been locked inside a candy shop, and I wrote it all down. As soon as the girl scampered off to the bathroom, I would start scribbling down notes. The edge of the bed or the corner of a table was my desk. I'd note down a good line, a sensual walk, a pained smile, all the details of life. Everything fascinated me. I wrote down everything that moved, and things never stopped moving, believe me. All around me, the world (the girl, the dress on the floor, my underwear lost in the sheets, that long naked back moving toward the stereo, then Bob Marley's music), the elements of my universe turned at top speed. How could words halt the flight of time, girls wheeling away, desire burning anew? Often I would fall asleep with my head against my old Remington, asking myself those unanswerable questions. Am I the troubadour of low-rent America, always on the edge of an overdose, up against the walls, handcuffs slapped on, with two cops breathing down my neck? America discounting her life, counting her pennies, the America of immigrants, blacks, and poor white girls who've lost their way? America of empty eyes and pallid dawn. In the end, I wrote that damned novel, and America was forced, as least as far as I was concerned, to come through on a few of her promises. I know she gives more to some than they need; with others, she swipes the hunk of stale bread from their clenched fists. But I made her pay at least a third of her debt. I'm naive, I know, I can see the audience smiling, but my mental system needs to believe in this victory, as tiny as it may be. A third of a victory. For others, not a penny of the debt has been paid. America owes an enormous amount to third world youth. I'm not just talking about historical debt (slavery, the rape of natural resources, the balance of payments, etc.), there's a sexual debt, too. Everything we've been promised by magazines, posters, the movies, television. America is a happy hunting ground, that's what gets beaten into our heads every day, come and stalk the most delicious morsels (young American beauties with long legs, pink mouths, superior smiles), come and pick the wild fruit of this new Promised Land. For you, young men of the third world, America will be a doe quivering under the buckshot of your caresses. The call went around the world, and we heard it, even the blue men of the desert heard it. Remember the global village? They've got American TV in the middle of the Sahara. Westward, ho! It was a new gold rush. And when each new arrival showed up, he was told, "Sorry, the party's over." I can still picture the sad smile of a Bedouin, old in years but still vigorous (remember, brother, those horny old goats from the Old Testament), who had sold his camel to attend the party. I met up with all of them in a tiny bar on Park Avenue. While you're waiting for the next fiesta, the Manpower counselor told us, you have to work. There's work for everyone in America (the old carrot and stick, brother). We've got you coming and going. What? Work? Our Bedouin didn't come here to work. He crossed the desert and sailed the seas because he'd been told that in America the girls were free and easy. Oh, no, you didn't quite understand! What didn't we understand from that showy sexuality, that profusion of naked bodies, that total disclosure, that Hollywood heat? You should know we have some very sophisticated devices in the desert; we can tune in America. The resolution is exceptional, and there's no interference in the Sahara. In the evening, we gather in our tents lit by the cathode screen and watch you. Watching how you do what you do is a great pleasure for us. Some pretty girl is always laughing on a beach somewhere. The next minute, a big blond guy shows up and jumps her. She slips between his fingers, and he chases her into the surf. She fights, but he holds her tight and both of them sink to the bottom. Every evening it's the same menu, with slight variations. The sea is bluer, the girls blonder, the guys more muscled. All our dreams revolve around this life of ease. That's what we want: the easy life. Those breasts and asses and teeth and laughter—after a while, it started affecting our libido. What could be more natural? And now, here we are in America, and you dare tell us that we didn't understand? Understand what? I ask the question again. What were we supposed to have understood? You made us mad with desire. Today, we stand before you, a long chain of men (in our country, adventure is the realm of men), penises erect, appetites insatiable, ready for the battle of the sexes and the races. We'll fight to the finish, America.

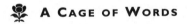

🌹 A CAGE OF WORDS

Joel Dreyfuss

I call it "the Phrase" and it comes up almost anytime Haiti is mentioned in the news: the Poorest Nation in the Western Hemisphere. These seven words represent a classic example of something absolutely true and absolutely meaningless at the same time.

On a recent trip to Haiti, I asked a young journalist working for an international news organization why the Phrase always appeared in her stories. "Even when I don't put it in," she confided, "the editors add it to the story."

The Phrase is a box, a metaphorical prison. If Haiti is the poorest country in the Western Hemisphere, that fact is supposed to place everything in context. Why we have such suicidal politics. Why we have such selfish politicians. Why we suffer so much misery. Why our people brave death on the high seas to wash up on the shores of Florida. After all, in this age where an advocacy of free markets is a substitute for foreign policy and Internet billionaires are created by the minute, being poor automatically makes you suspect. You must have some moral failing, some fatal flaw, some cultural blindness to not be prosperous. And what applies to the individual also applies to entire countries.

In my parents' generation, more than a few middle-class Haitians tried to deny that poverty back home was so prevalent. When I heard older Haitians stammer and object to the characterization, I wondered if they were trying to put Haiti's best foot forward, or just trying to convince themselves. Of course, the poverty was not always as obvious as it is now, having moved from the countryside into Port-au-Prince so that it spills into the main thoroughfares and the fashionable neighborhoods. Too many of us *Dyasporas*, having the advantage of distance to confront the truths of Haiti, would not even consider denying the desperate state of our poor brethren.

But the Phrase still grates with us because it also denies so much else about Haiti: our art, our music, our rich Afro-Euro-American culture. It denies the humanity of Haitians, the capacity to survive, to overcome, even to triumph over this poverty, a historical experience we share with so many other in this same Western Hemisphere. The Second American Invasion cast a harsh media spotlight on Haiti. The first black republic got more attention from the powerful news organizations of the West than it ever had in its history. But that scrutiny was ultimately disappointing. We learned once again that coverage is not the same as understanding. The Phrase became an easy out for reporters confronting the complexities they could barely begin to plumb. What a difference it would have been if American, or French, or British journalists had looked through the camera at their audience and declared, "Yes, this is a poor country, but like Ireland or Portugal, it has also produced great art. Yes, this poor country has suffered brutal government and yet, like Russia or Brazil, it has produced great writers and scholars. Yes, many of Haiti's most downtrodden, like the Jews in America or the Palestinians in the Middle East, have fled and achieved more success in exile than they ever would at home." Such statements would have linked Haiti to the rest of the world. They would have made it seem less mysterious, less unsolvable, less exotic. But then, that really wasn't the purpose of most reporting about Haiti over the last few years. Keeping the veil over the island was easier than trying to understand factions and divisions and mistrust and history. And it gave America an out if the intervention failed. So foreign journalists fell back on the Phrase. It was shorthand. It was neat. And it told the world nothing about Haiti that it didn't already know.

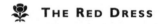

🌸 THE RED DRESS

Patricia Benoît

1982. TV. The nightly news. Bodies on the beach, faces behind barbed wire. Any one of them could be related to me. Rudolph Giuliani, then assistant attorney general of the United States, now New York City mayor, finger wagging: we have no problem with refugees as long as they come by the proper channels: (Rude refugees. Bad refugees. *Ça ne se fait pas*, it's just not done to come by boat and die on U.S. beaches). These refugees are economic, not political. There are no human-rights abuses in Haiti.

I want to break the television.

What about the women, men, and children who died fighting for freedom? What about my father, imprisoned then released and lucky enough to escape before the *macoutes* came for him again and lucky enough to get asylum and bring us out by the proper channels twenty years ago? I get tired of yelling and decide to do something.

The United States government transforms an abandoned building into a detention center in Brooklyn's former Navy Yard. After much political wrangling, a group of activist priests, themselves exiled by the Duvalier dictatorship, are finally allowed to organize English classes in the center.

I start teaching in one of those January winters so hard on island

people. It is an out-of-the-way place, a group of abandoned industrial buildings not far from the Brooklyn Bridge, several high-
way overpasses, and a housing project. The streets are almost
empty.

A hundred women and men live in this red building with windows covered with dirt and wire mesh. Black and Latino guards have
been hired especially for the occasion. After the guard at the door
inspects the contents of my bag, he flashes a smile and reprises with
perfect comic timing the refrain of a television commercial: "Welcome to Roach Motel. Roaches check in but they don't check out."
Humor as a weapon against a dirty job?

The men and women have been separated into different parts of
the building and are not allowed to see each other. There is no yard,
no place for physical activity or even a short walk in the sun.

When I start, they have been there for two months. They will
end up spending more than a year without ever going out, except
for the rare authorized medical or legal appointment.

After I pass inspection I wait as several guards bring the women
out of the "living" area, one by one, through a metal door. There
are about twenty of them, many in their twenties like me, none
older than fifty, all waiting impatiently to get on with their lives.
This must be a special occasion, a break in the monotony, for the
women make the most of the secondhand clothing donated through
the Haitian priests. They dress impeccably. No pants; only dresses,
skirts and blouses, pretty and demure as if for church. The youngest,
barely out of their teens, highlight their youth and beauty with perfect makeup and brightly painted nails.

I am not allowed into the living area, but later the women tell
me that there are dormitories with bunk beds, guards everywhere,
and a common room with the television always on. The windows
are so dirty they can barely see outside. Where are we? What is this

place? Nothing to do except watch TV. No family to take care of. No meals to cook. They miss their husbands and boyfriends, and relatives and friends who are on the other side of these walls and on the other side of the sea. Six months later, one of their lawyers argues unsuccessfully to at least let them have rice and beans instead of hot dogs and canned food.

Class is in a room with fluorescent lighting, no windows, and a guard at the door. I teach but I also ask for help with my *Kreyòl*. My pronunciation is bad. I make mistakes. They laugh. We laugh together. This helps narrow the gulf between us: my twenty years of exile.

A face, an expression, a gesture reminds me of an aunt, a friend, my grandmother. Do you need anything? I ask.

They give me letters to send back home to worrying relatives and dictate a list of hair products. I stuff the letters into my shoulder bag and take them to the post office. I feel useful.

The night before class, I transfer hair relaxers and pomades from their forbidden glass containers (glass shards as a way out?) into plastic ones.

As the Latina guard carefully examines the containers and their messy contents, she finally blurts out: They have so many donations! People have given them so much, so many boxes, we have to put them in special storage! Looks at me like I'm stupid, like I've been had, taken by people already getting so much for free. They have so much, she says. Doesn't she know about divide and conquer? Setting the have-little against the have-not? Doesn't she know they—we— are the descendants of Toussaint and Dessalines, who led the only successful slave uprising in the history of the world and defeated Napoleon's troops and founded the first black republic? She probably doesn't even think I'm Haitian.

I want to narrow the gap. I am lucky. They are unlucky. Accidents of birth. I give out my home phone number in case of emergencies. I hesitate slightly before I do, fearing a deluge of phone calls, but days pass and no one calls, until Philocia. She is one of the youngest, distracted and hesitant whenever I ask her a question, not one of my best students.

Please, she says, can you do something for me?

Of course, I say, worried by her sudden assertiveness.

Well, Valentine's Day is coming and next Friday there is going to be a party and they are going to let us see the men. I am going to see my boyfriend—so I need a dress.

A dress? I ask. Maybe I haven't heard right.

Yes, she says. A red dress. Size eight.

I look through my closet as if a red dress might miraculously appear. This is not what I had in mind when I gave out my number. Didn't I say in case of an emergency?

I call a friend. A red dress? she asks.

Yes.

Red for hearts and roses?

I guess.

Have any of the other women asked for dresses?

No.

Her reaction convinces me not to ask anyone else. This one frivolous request I am sure will make the other refugees look bad, make people think that Giuliani is right after all, that they have just come here for economic advantages, that they have come here to shop.

I go to the clothing stores in my East Village neighborhood. No red dress in sight, and certainly no dress that I could imagine her ever wanting to wear. Too funky and outrageous, nothing her style. Besides, what if I do find one? I don't even have a real job. She must think I'm rich. Maybe the guard was right, maybe I'm being had.

Two days before the party, I take Philocia aside. I'm sorry, I say, but I couldn't find a red dress. I tried, but it's not easy. She smiles sweetly. I look down at her carefully manicured nails and think someone must have donated red nail polish to go with the dress she won't be wearing. Thank you, she says, *mèsi*, like someone used to not getting what she wants. Why couldn't she have asked for something serious, something vital and important? Then I would have done anything!

Valentine's Day has come and gone. We are in the middle of class when Jeanne, an attentive, serious student, a woman in her forties, a *madansara* who used to sell pots and pans in the market of Jacmel, starts to cry.

What's wrong? someone asks.

What's wrong, Jeanne? I ask.

More tears. Silence. She rocks herself gently, back and forth.

I can't stand it anymore, she says, I want to go back home.

But they will kill you if you go back, someone says.

I don't care. I want to die in my country like a *moun,* like a person, not here like a dog.

More silence. I hand her a tissue. Are they all thinking the same thing?

Now, I say, surprised at the authority of my voice, this is what they want. They want to wear you down, so that you will go back and tell the others and they will be afraid to come.

More silence. What is Jeanne thinking? What are they all thinking?

Then, from the back of the room, a small still voice.

Not me.

It is Philocia of the red dress. *Mwen mem.* I will never go back. I don't care what they do to me. I spent two days in the water holding on to a piece of wood from the boat. There were dead people all around me. I'm not going back.

I look at her and she has not moved. I realize that she has never left the water and that I have understood nothing.

Now I want to find her a dress in every possible shade of red . . . for roses . . . for hearts . . . red for the blood of Toussaint and Dessalines flowing in her veins.

Something in the Water . . . Reflections of a People's Journey

Nikòl Payen

The windowed door of my hospital room framed scurrying white uniforms. Inside, the silence of isolation left plenty of time for interior monologues. The medication and its lingering scent made my head fuzzy and paralyzed my tongue. My spirit seemed to be having difficulty catching up with my body, like the distorted windshield view of a rainstormed road. I anxiously waited to see whether or not this physician would corroborate my overseas diagnosis of bronchial asthma, which was beginning to seem mild now that I was up against possible heavy hitters like tuberculosis, PCP pneumonia, and HIV.

Lying there, I could almost see my dad's concerned face, his eyes widening as his deep, stern voice prepared me with Haitian proverbs, tales about our clan, warnings and cautions for my work at Guantánamo Bay. Most important, however, was his promise of ancestral protection. So off I went, surrounded by my invisible army.

The IV stand was beginning to feel like an awkward extension of my anatomy, contributing to my claustrophobia. As I lay there, I struggled to pinpoint exactly when and why my body broke down. Was it the night-and-day contrast in temperature? Days with temperatures that sometimes sent boa constrictors, iguanas, and banana rats looking for shelter under my cot, then onto the clothes that dangled from my partially open dufflebag. At times the leftover wind from the Windward Passage would stir up the baked sand, lashing my face or filling my nose and mouth with grit. Or perhaps it was the cobalt-blue, diamond-lit evening sky that would seduce me into rolling up the sides of the tent, allowing the night's chilling vapors to invade my lungs.

Time was strangely distorted on that mound of land—days long, nights short, and mornings difficult to embrace. I could always set my watch, though, by the chants of exercising soldiers that began with the 5 a.m. dosage of pesticide the military used to wage the war against bugs. When it was kind, the fumes tickled inside your nostrils. Otherwise, you went into a choking cough that could rage for twenty minutes.

Before three days could come and go, my life had undergone a complete metamorphosis. *Kreyòl*, the language whose purpose in my life up until now had been to pain and confuse me, would prove an asset. It became my passport to the American-occupied naval base in Guantánamo Bay, Cuba. The Justice Department would use me as a medium—or, as my contract stipulated, an interpreter—to execute its mission. Haitians fleeing political persecution—unleashed by a coup d'état that had overthrown Haiti's first democratically elected president, Jean-Bertrand Aristide—were being detained while they awaited interviews for political asylum.

I was one of sixteen language specialists. We worked in a defunct airplane hangar, freshly painted white, which held about fourteen thousand people when full. The scent of sweaty bodies thickened the already damp air. Their united sound of confused chatter echoed from the hollow interior, creating a dense hum of marketplace conversation. Bodies lay in rows on olive-green cots, all their worldly possessions on the concrete floor beside them—clothes, shoes, personal documents, in black plastic garbage bags or homemade straw sacks.

I rode the yellow school bus that transported service people through the camp. It was my means of getting to work as well. On the days when I arrived at the bus stop early, I would sit on a wooden park bench while an awakening sun pierced my sunglasses. All too often, the bath I had taken in insect repellent proved fruitless as last night's rainfall summoned what seemed like the island's entire mosquito population to feast on my exposed arms and legs. Waiting impatiently, I waved off a buzzing bee that had grown tired of a sugar-coated bottle neck from a nearby steel-grid garbage can. In the distance, a topless green army truck appeared, hauling soldiers to work. The overcrowded vehicle screeched at the red light, burying us in a fog of dust.

While I hadn't any preconceived notions about the architectural layout of a military base, never had I imagined it to be so elaborate—an actual replication of a city, a setup I suspect to be crucial in setting the underlining tone for the severity and intensity of the military training process. Like any other American town, it had a post office, a bank, a church, a gas station, credit union, firehouse, schools, hospital, restaurants, a 7-Eleven, a mall, and even a McDonald's. The neighborhoods seemed lifted directly from a suburban blueprint onto the desert landscape, the houses bearing prefabricated faces reminiscent of small towns in upstate New York. But even with the skeletal details of everyday life surrounding them, Guantánamo remained a wall-less prison.

I had committed to memory the entire bus route, which was easy to do. We would ride past Treasures & Trivia, a thrift store operated by civilian wives to occupy their day while their husbands worked.

Up the hill brought us to the Jamaican Club, an after-hours spot where contracted Jamaican workers earning below minimum wage convened to bond and essentially keep sane amidst the sterility. We careened around the corner to a port and picked up a few more sailors who seemed anxious to get to their destination.

As usual, the day seemed innocent until we pulled into the ferry landing—the stop before mine. Like clockwork my stomach knotted and my heart pounded against my chest, asking to be let out. Winding around the final hill, we passed the grandest edifice on the island—the Pink Palace, the military's administrative headquarters, strategically planted on top of the hill overlooking the entire camp. This was where most of the important meetings were held by high-ranking military officials to plan and strategize with their Washington counterparts. The bus gave a final jerk indicating the end of its route.

Each day found me unprepared to digest the misery and despair that awaited me at the gate. Going back in there day after day seemed pointless, attempting to nurse physical and emotional wounds that I could not yet fully comprehend, let alone heal.

"A boat of forty-five was intercepted last night near the Windward Passage," was my substitute morning greeting from my supervisor. This tidbit was sure to structure much of the day's work. The voyage almost always promised an illness of some sort, followed by the culture shock of camp conditions. Sometimes the newcomers' eyes were weary, hazed by dehydration and seasickness. Some were badly sunburned, some wore big grins, usually a sign of relief at having been spared the swallow of the ocean. Others were generally happy about the possibilities that awaited them. After exchanging greetings and tips from familiar faces from the same or neighboring towns, the newcomers awaited the formal unveiling of their new reality. Sometimes the camp provided a ground for family reunification. When they arrived—some barefoot and meagerly attired, others clad in church-wear of sequined, taffeta dresses—they were taken to Camp Alpha, where the processing began. Hours would pass before they could all be photographed, fingerprinted, and given identification cards.

Fighting the fierce sunrays, children hopped about, alternating feet to keep their soles from burning on the cooked tar. Colonies of flies comfortably rested on their choice of heads and faces of those awaiting the final step: acquisition of an ID bracelet, marked with a bar code similar to those found on the side of household products. Some days, this long ritual—the stamping of the refugees with the marks of ownership—accounted for an entire workday. The refugees were happy to find *Kreyòl* speakers among the processing staff. I often walked around continuously answering any questions, explaining the ensuing immigration procedures, tending to those who were ill, and troubleshooting for anything from diapers to emergency-room arrangements and anything in between.

Feeding time introduced the newcomers to the dietary convenience of the Western world—packaged food, a first for many. They curiously deciphered the contents of their brown plastic "Meals Ready to Eat," or MREs. Some ate ravenously, while others whose palates could not make an instant adjustment to the foreign taste eagerly passed on their unused rations to unsated neighbors. Sometimes they were used for bartering. The box of chicken à la king, stroganoff, and beef stew, a favorite among the brave, contained all the components of a well-thought-out meal: an entree, instant beverages, condiments, and for dessert, various junk foods, M&M's the most popular. The military often complained of the haughtiness of Haitians. How dare they criticize perfectly delicious war-ready meals?

Creative survival instincts blossomed before my eyes under less than favorable conditions, unfolding a culture. The women converted sheets into Sunday dresses, while the men went as far as creating a radio station from transistor radios given to them by the military. The two most memorable parts of the day, as in the hospital, were mealtimes and visiting hours. The neighboring camps were also established communities. As the families were scattered throughout, visitation rights were sometimes granted. While the women cooked, cleaned, washed, nurtured the children, and carried on the traditions, the men created furniture and paintings, took in a game of soccer, cards, or dominoes, or circularly discussed politics. Conversations were stimulated by their current isolated condition as well as the Miami-based Haitian *Kreyòl* radio broadcast, *Voix de L'Amérique*— the only outside news to penetrate the wall-less penitentiary. Even the children created dolls, toys, puppets, boats, trains, planes. I marveled at an ability they took for granted.

Unfortunately the tragedies were equally colorful. The camp was nearly hit by a cyclone; three hundred and fifty people drowned trying to escape to "Castro's" Cuba to see if communism could offer a kinder hand.

When the glare of the sun, the chaos of the camp, and the rhetoric became overwhelming, I walked long and hard, away from everything as far away as possible, though never far enough. On one such occasion I escaped to the bathroom, located in a neighboring hangar. Halfway to my destination, the glare of the sun reflected off a steel cage, immediately attracting me. I walked toward the object, sinking into the cooked tar of the gummy pavement with each step. Encaged, a seven-year-old boy sat listlessly playing with a pair of broken flip-flops. "A soldier put me here because when I went to eat I kept getting pushed from the food line," explained the boy. "He said I was making trouble, so I have to sit here until I learn my lesson. Can you get me some water, Miss?" High up, a guard sat post in a twenty-foot tower equipped with a rifle, a gun, binoculars, and a video camera. He recorded my interaction while adjusting his walkie-talkie.

The sun hid behind a darkening stratus cloud, transmitting an orange-yellow tint that hovered over the entire island. The bus took the dusty route to my living quarters. The glow of a setting sun outlined the smoke of floating dust left by the tires. I usually liked to linger in the camp after hours, when things began to settle and the true culture of the environment surfaced, transcending the cohesion of the makeshift community, but that day I was anxious to leave on time. At a distance, a caterpillar of soldiers clad in white T-shirts and gray shorts getting in their mandatory evening exercise swerved by, their chanting fading as the distance between us widened. As the bus pulled up near my barrack, I made a quick run for it. Walking through a patch of swamp land, a swarm of fruit fly-like insects took cover in my ears, eyes and mouth. It was nearly seven and I hoped to complete my cooking and laundry.

McCalla was a small city. Each day I took a twenty-minute ferry ride from Leeward, where I lived, to the Windward side of the island, where I worked. The ride was awkward and always reminded me of my outsider status. Some days the 7 a.m. ferry was filled to capacity: I would be sandwiched between servicemen, which I hated, or have to stand by the rail for the entire ride. As much as I loved the view of the water and the wind gently stroking my face, these visions of serenity were eclipsed by my own paranoia. The ferry seats reminded me of church pews and some mornings they were equally precious, as I tried to get the last twenty minutes of sleep. Sometimes, I resorted to sitting in the compartment under the deck. The ferry also transported large trucks and machinery to the work side of the island. When we docked, the machinery backed off the lower deck first. The sailor in charge then hand-signaled for passengers from the top deck to single-file off the craft. Once on the ferry landing, we'd wait for the bus that took us to work. Some mornings, time permitting, we procrastinated, putting off going into the camp by stopping at McDonald's and picking up a high-sodium, nutritionally unsound breakfast. I often found myself gobbling down a sausage McSomething or Another not for any reason other than to reconnect me to home, where such rubbish would never touch my lips.

One night on the last ferry with two other translators returning from a party from the Windward side to our living quarters on the Leeward side, I discovered the strategic design of the island. A man's eyes rolled back in his head after he vomited uncontrollably. Panic-stricken, the other translator screamed at him questions of concern, while I quickly alerted the driver to our crisis. He pushed some odd buttons that made strange noises and in two minutes, like a scene from *Batman*, a secret tunnel produced a motor raft that transported us to the principal naval hospital. This, complemented by the acres of land mines strategically plotted throughout the burned grass partitioned by steel fences with barbed-wire topping, a deterrent for Cubans who were curious about democracy, not the ones who crossed the border every morning to work for the U.S. government, left me in awe of the island's intricate readiness for war. The chopping of helicopters was a familiar noise, as was the arbitrary explosion of cannons. The twenty-four-hour guard towers reassured both sides protection of their respective countries. Sun up to sundown, soldiers stood guard at the borders with their guns permanently aimed in the direction of the enemy.

That morning found me fussing with the contents of my knapsack, trying to get to some important notes from a recent meeting. Dashing in late to the eight-thirty meeting already under way, I arrived in time for the tail end of a heated debate about the nutritional value of the meals fed to refugees. These meetings were, for the most part, a waste of time because no one intended to rectify any wrongdoing; not really. So far as I could gather, the interpreters' meetings were held for sheer appeasement, an answer to our complaints of exclusion from the seven o'clock meetings with high-ranking government officials and asylum officers.

Today's hot debate was centered on a memo warning us against fraternizing with the "migrants," an offense that would not go unpunished. The list was long in its definition and examples of fraternizing were thoroughly spelled out, so there would be no misunderstandings. The content of the memo was the end result of yet another recent problem. It was rumored that military personnel and interpreters were beginning to establish intimate relationships with some of the migrants and the purchase of luxury items such as shampoo, conditioners, permanents, hair grease, and in some instances clothes on their behalf, was proof of this foul act. I was particularly embarrassed when one interpreter was caught on video accepting money from the migrants in exchange for a definite place on the next plane to Miami—a promise he was unauthorized to make.

Near my assignment's end, repatriation offered a free ride to refugees who had failed to prove a "credible fear" of persecution and were consequently to be returned to Haiti. I reluctantly volunteered to accompany them back. Though the two-day journey promised to be a grueling experience, I was prepared to make any sacrifice to return to my homeland after fifteen years of unintended absence.

It cost the U.S. approximately one million dollars per day to run the camp, and each repatriation neared $100,000, so filling the cutter to capacity was a must before we could be on our way. I arrived at the pier to find three other ships, housing a total of fifteen hundred refugees, ready to leave. We were scheduled for a 9 a.m. departure but were running late. On a good day, the deck fit five hundred bodies comfortably, if they were aligned sardine-style. Our ship housed only two hundred people on board, thus the holdup. Six-and-a-half hours later, with only fifty bodies added to the count, we were given clearance to leave so as to avoid an evening departure, when the ferocity of the Windward Passage would peak. I was escorted to my two-by-four cabin, which I believed to belong to some high-ranking officer. It offered me the privilege of a private bathroom half the size of the room. A pinup of Kathy Ireland graced the tiny closet door. A navy-blue jumpsuit, the only visible item of clothing, dangled solo in the darkness.

As the only civilian and the only woman working on the U.S. *Escanaba*, a Coast Guard cutter—the steel shark that guarded our national "security" in the form of international "drug busts"—I was at everyone's disposal twenty-four hours a day and partly responsible for maintaining order on board, whatever happened. En route, clandestine discussions held by the refugees and me in the camp were openly voiced here on the ship. Both the refugees and I found comfort in our mutual distrust of the asylum process. I had often overheard conversations corroborating these allegations from higher-ups. Programmed to spit out whatever numbers Washington entrusted them to produce that day in the name of efficiency and a job well done, these functionaries lost neither sleep nor appetite over the desperate accounts of a people whose destiny lay in their hands. "How are those numbers coming along?" was the question of the day, every day.

I remember being told the story of one twelve-year-old boy from Cité-Soleil: He was so thin that a thumb and index finger alone could have encircled his thigh. With tears rimming his eyes, he fought to keep from crying as he explained his dilemma. After the coup, his father had gone out to search for oil. When his father failed to return, his mother sent him out to search for his father and instead he found his father's corpse. He finally made it home, only to find his mother riddled with bullets, murdered by soldiers seeking revenge on democracy supporters. His family supported Lavalas, the people's movement, and for that he was wanted by the authorities.

Then there were two teenage girls, stocky, angry, and confused by the unexpected turn of events that left their lives upside down. It was as if someone had scrambled up a puzzle and asked them to fix it. They complained nonstop, frustrated by their inability to see what stared them right in the face. "I'm going to kill myself," one said. "What do I have ahead of me? I'm not going to Miami despite the fact that the Section Chief killed my parents in front of me. The only reason I was spared rape was because I had my period. I managed to get on a boat, and now I'm returning to the hell I thought was behind me." Though she put on a tough exterior, I told her to reverse it and to let her toughness flow from inside. This would enable her to better deal with life's unexpected blows. The human spirit is so resilient, its elasticity often surprised me, I told her enthusiastically. So far as I was concerned, she had already dealt with the most difficult part. But then again, I was merely speculating. I suppose I'll never know for certain from what she fled nor exactly what awaited her. "But that's all God's business isn't it?" I said. She smiled.

Dinner calmed everyone down somewhat. All concerns, needs, and worries finally began to drift with the fading day. Hours later when the sun made way for the moon and the stars, the chaos of the day began to subside, as did the buzzing of those returning home. No longer were there conversations about hypocrisy, distrust, and injustice. All had come to accept that which was most dreaded— returning home. There was a hush now, the ferocity of the clouds and the strength of the wind had calmed everyone's frustration and demanded silence.

Some time during the dark morning I was awakened by frantic pounding on my cabin door. It was one of the soldiers, breathlessly ordering me to tend to an emergency. He disappeared long before I could become coherent enough to ask for an explanation. I made my way up the tiny steel staircase, to find a robust fifteen-year-old unaccompanied minor under restraint, the girl I had been consoling that afternoon. It required the strength of three men to hold down this poor child convulsing in a screaming fit. Finally, she was pinned flat on her stomach while another serviceman tied her feet together. Two sailors simultaneously struggled to handcuff her hands behind her back as a fellow Haitian was instructed to hold her head fixed to one side.

We were entering the mouth of the Windward Passage. The wind fiercely rocked our vessel while lightning illuminated the dark, angry sky. Roaring thunder drowned my conversations, pulling rain from the clouds and pouring it over our bodies. This outburst caused some to grumble explanations of a jilted lover, others claimed her insanity came by way of a hex from the other woman. As she went in and out of piranha-like biting fits, a thinly built, gray-haired, mild-mannered man from the girl's native town of Jérémie accounted for her epileptic history. She had been fine for both his and my conversation of earlier that day. It seemed that the young lady I had tried to dissuade from suicide had manifested these feelings after all. Eventually she was subdued with her hand and foot securely tied to a pole on the flight deck. Lightning ripped across the sky and spotlighted her crucified shadow followed by the sky's disapproving grumble. I wrapped her in a wool blanket to shield her from the wind.

What was to have been a two-day voyage turned into a week of drifting in the Atlantic between Haiti and Cuba, in preparation to intercept incoming refugees even before the ink on President Bush's newly imposed executive order could fully dry. My trek through the Middle Passage dragged me through the murky road of history, determined to make me feel a pain that was centuries deep and supposedly resolved. Yet this nightmare gnawed so deep within me, not even my assimilationist lifestyle could mitigate it.

Witnessing two hundred fifty bodies enroped in slave-ship fashion on deck to be baked by the summer blaze or soaked by impulsive skies if nature willed left me feeling helpless and uneasy. We seemed to be going backward—in time—in history. But time spoke softly, gently unveiling its truth before me. The pieces of my parents' past, which they had difficulty talking about, were gladly exhibited through the troubled spirits of those who sat before me to translate their perplexities. An Abyssinian-looking beauty sat before me complaining about the factory where she worked sewing bras. A mandatory eighteen-hour day with no lunch and no break except those to fight off advances by her boss who promised her, in return, a raise of fifteen cents per hour. But this was mild compared to the threats of death received by her husband, whose goat had wandered off into a section chief's yard and fed on his garden. Or the woman whose community group was plastered with photos of a rooster and Aristide, thereby making her a candidate for death. Young men complained that Haiti was so plagued politically that their congregation for any reason, even for church, left them suspect of political activities. Or the tailor who was commissioned to make clothes for the sister of a certain section chief who, disagreeing with the asking price of her new dress, sicced her brother on him. Others reached the camp by happenstance, as one gentleman explained that he'd been fishing and fell asleep.

I'll never forget my first reintroduction to Haiti. We were nearing the pier when a refugee pointed to Gonaives, and Port-de-Paix, up north. "There's Môle Saint Nicolas," exclaimed a young man, proudly explaining the century-old U.S. desire to construct a military base there. This would be strategically ideal since Cuba and Jamaica, the other two largest countries occupying the Caribbean basin, are a stone's throw away. The fog revealed a sketch of our intended destination, the ship chaplain pointed to Sacré Coeur, a century-old landmark church. I gazed in disbelief, reflecting vaguely on the times when this cathedral served as the ultimate sanctuary for me and my family for Sunday mass some two decades ago.

The refugees were instructed to return their yellow I.D. cards, at last relieved from the tight wrist-squeezing of plastic bar-coded bracelets. Their curiosity about what lay ahead provided an occasion for me to give a briefing outlining the final phase of the procedure. At the wharf they were met by Red Cross personnel, sometimes accompanied by U.S. Embassy officials, who dealt with politically complex cases. The returnees were given an exit interview and fifteen Haitian dollars, which many claimed was insufficient for their long journey home. That day, the string of armed Haitian military officials awaiting their disembarkation left many fearful for their lives. Panic was lent validity by concerns about being followed home by the same would-be attackers who had been responsible for their initial departure. The U.S. military promised safety, but even if they hadn't, the Haitians had no means to negotiate. So they halfheartedly, yet peacefully, disembarked. When the ship was nearly vacant, I caught a U.S. State Department staff member handing the bag of I.D. cards to Haitian soldiers. Confused and frustrated, I looked for an ally until it dawned on me that no one on board remotely shared my concern.

On the return trip, the calm night sky twinkled on the ocean while angry phosphorescent waters pounded at the ship from bow to stern.

The ordeal cast me into a four-day bout with insomnia. Even the ocean, hard as she tried, was unable to cradle me to sleep. For each night while they weathered the cold winds on deck, I wrestled with the displaced faces that haunted me in my cabin while I lay nestled in wool blankets. With their concerns and uncertainties etched deeply into their faces, strong and tired eyes imposed inquisitive gazes, looking for answers I also sought.

Meanwhile, back in the captain's dining room I began wondering to what I owed the honor of past-life luxuries—cloth napkins, sterling silver flatware, and china actually used and not only displayed. And waiters, four waiters who stood post on each corner of the table, eager to tend to the captain's every need. The quality and size of one's portions matched one's rank. Contrary to the migrants' restricted diets food flowed nonstop in the forms of soup, salad, entree, dessert, coffee, followed by the point of the dinner invitation. The closing conversation was to get an assessment of my personal limitations regarding the perils of my assignment. In other words, to size up the distance I would go for my people and my two countries, one that had my allegiance as a birthright, the other hoping to win it.

Despite the hazardous duty conditions, which had already claimed the life of one interpreter, I volunteered to be lowered by rope from the cutter into a tiny motor raft in an attempt to negotiate with prospective refugees on behalf of the United States government. Looking at the flimsy craft in the middle of the hungry, shark-infested waters, I felt the pressure of pleading to win their confidence as their boat repeatedly threatened to capsize. The sun began its descent and my sneakers were soaked from the puddle that collected in our motor boat. One of the teenage boys leaned on the bow. Their ragged sail was tied to the flimsy pole that struggled to hold it. "Why should I go on the ship, why should I trust you?" asked a dark-skinned man in his early twenties, turning up his nose as if he literally smelled something foul. I was lost for an adequate response except, *I'm all you've got here and you have to believe in my good intentions.* And besides, I was unprepared to watch them drown.

The mother wore only the bottom half of what used to be a dress, her shriveled sagging breasts dangled lifelessly against her badly scarred body. With dark spots and welts all over her back, her hair was ravaged and she spoke in delirium, a blur. "My sister, my baby," she muttered. Each time she tried to express herself, she was unable to add any more information to where she had left off. "My aunt and her baby were with us on the boat, the baby became ill. She plunged in the ocean with the baby saying she could no longer stand the suffering," explained the young man. "She's not good in her head," he finished.

They appeared to be badly dehydrated and said that they had not had water in three days. A colony of flies and insects buzzed around the stale vomit that floated atop the semi-flooded boat. Apparently they had been "maroons," on the run, for several months, living in caves, traveling underground by night, surviving on coconuts and wild berries. By the grace of people in the various towns, eventually they were able to escape. A *vèvè* of Agwe, the water god, decorated the mint-green craft. They had christened it *"Kris Kapab,"* or "Christ Can," inscribed in blood-red paint.

The father was a fisherman, his gentleness reflected in his overall demeanor. "Do you have medicine on the ship?" inquired the fiery youth, who seemed to be reconsidering the idea of coming on board. He showed me the colony of parasites, white wormlike ones that had been eating away at his brother's scalp for the past few months. I looked at the visible rise in the puddle and as the boat dipped backwards, I quickly blurted, "Yes." I was getting tired, my mouth was dry, there were eighteen of them and only one of me and I didn't know how much longer I could sustain a coherent argument. The youth, who seemed to be the head negotiator, the city-slicker type, needing one final push, began to look as if he believed me, so said his eyes and his face. I looked at his Nelson Mandela T-shirt and asked how he thought the character on his shirt would handle this particular dilemma. This was the clincher. Mandela had become a universal living icon for courage, strength, persistence, and faith.

After three hours of intense creative negotiations catalyzed by the spell of an intensely beautiful set of almond-shaped eyes belonging to an eight-year-old refugee girl, I finally convinced this mistrustful family to come on board. A conspiratorial chill raced through me as I watched their craft along with all their worldly possessions set afire, a ritual that branded a mental scar on these victims and on me. It seemed a sacrilegious act for which we all would be punished.

The ocean danced and curtsied. Once again the empty ship was filled with laughter and jokes. For many, the last forty-eight hours had been a mere incident that would forever vanish into nothingness. Its effect on me, at that point, was apparent in emotions only, like the sharp pain that registers that a finger has been burned. It is not until days later, when the wounded area darkens, that the effect actually becomes visible. Astonished by the turn of events, I could only think, "Did this really just happen? Was I partly responsible for someone's impending death?" The thought horrified me. Sitting in a corner, I reflected quietly on the faces, the stories, and the concerns, however remote, that had taken precedence over my own needs, even if only for a short time.

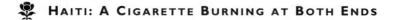 Haiti: A Cigarette Burning at Both Ends

Marie Ketsia Théodore-Pharel

On August 31, 1987, the last day of summer vacation, I got up early to go to Filene's Basement to shop for school clothes with my mother. I was twelve years old. We got off the T at Park Street near the Boston State House so my mother could make a stop at the bank. As we walked out of the train station, we were stopped by fire trucks and police barricades holding onlookers at bay. Above the streets loomed the highest steps of the Boston State House, still soaked and blackened by what seemed like a badly sprayed swastika. With a closer look, I saw that it was a man, burned to a grotesque crisp so that the most visible part of him now were his scorched legs, the unbending knees raised toward the sky. We asked what had happened and were told that he was a Haitian man who had soaked himself in gasoline, lit a match, and set himself on fire. His name was Antoine Thurel and he was fifty-six years old. The only clue to why he had killed himself was a large placard on which he had written a final letter in French. Loosely translated the sign read in part, "Because of many difficulties and my family and religious responsibilities, I want to offer myself in holocaust for the complete liberation of my country. . . . May Haiti live for the new liberation."

Like the heroes of centuries past, like Boukman, Toussaint,

83

Christophe, and Dessalines, and all the others who had given their lives fighting for the "liberation" of our country, Mr. Thurel had made the ultimate sacrifice. He had proven that not all men go to war because they are forced to, but some because they feel they must set an example, sacrifice themselves in order to incite all of us to change. *Koupe tèt, boule kay*, was the war cry of our ancestors. "Cut off heads and burn houses," starting with all that is most precious to us, our houses, our temples, our bodies. In a foreign country, on foreign soil, Antoine Thurel had given his life for a never-ending quest for freedom, not only his own but all of ours.

The day Mr. Thurel died, as I watched the spot where his body burned again on the six o'clock news, I thought of one of the last sayings of an old man whom I called "Père" who lived with my family. Père was a quiet, reserved man who analyzed everything; he was one of the brains who fled Haiti during the Sixties' brain-drain. Before he died of old age, in exile, Père had uttered a phrase which I would not completely understand for years.

"Haiti is a cigarette burning at both ends," he had said.

In their own way, both Père and Antoine Thurel could have been alluding to Edna St. Vincent Millay's poem "First Fig" about living fast, dying young, and leaving a beautiful corpse.

> My candle burns at both ends;
> It will not last the night;
> but ah, my foes, and oh, my friends—
> It gives a lovely light.

Still, I found Père's metaphor troubling. Is this why Mr. Thurel had died, for a cigarette burning at both ends? The imagery of a hopeless country being destroyed was one more to add to my list of negative things that I, as a Haitian child—and now a Haitian woman

and mother—had been told about Haiti, about myself, not by out-
siders but by my own. Mr. Thurel's action and Père's words made
me wonder about my love for Haiti and my love for myself as a
Haitian.

Haitians don't trust each other.

Haitian families, whether they know it or not, teach self-hatred.
I grew up with plenty of self-denigrating idioms, proverbs that offered such advice as: Don't let any Haitian boy touch the center of
your palm; he'll steal your decency and turn you into a trollop. Don't
let anyone read your books; they'll find whatever blessing was there
for you. Don't eat from anyone; they'll steal your *bonanj*, your good
angel. Don't study with others; they'll steal your intelligence. Safeguard your underwear because people could hurt your chances of
having children. "*Depi nan Ginen, nèg te rayi nèg,*" even in Africa,
blacks hated each other. At first I thought this distrusting advice was
part of my own family's proverbs, but I noticed that many of my
Haitian friends also cautiously lived by these same rules.

It wasn't until I went to live in Cameroon, Africa, that I realized
that blacks in Africa and elsewhere did love each other as a rule and
that those who hated one another were exceptions to that rule. Only
when we were paired against one another in divide-and-conquer
style did that hatred begin. This love was reaffirmed for me by my
host family in Cameroon. Sleeping in the same bed with my host
sisters, I felt a kind of peace I had never felt before in my life. I felt
like a tiger cub resting beside her mother's belly. I still feel that
warmth and love when I receive a nod or an acknowledging smile
from a black person or a Haitian person in the streets of Boston,
New York, or Miami. But according to the proverbs and idioms
that we are taught, we are all supposed to hate each other.

Haiti is a woman with two sets of children.

I have always been told and have come to realize for myself that

Haiti *is* like a woman with two sets of children, the elite and the masses. The elite are the children born to luxury, in wedlock, and the masses are the children born to poverty, the bastards. The elites abuse or completely neglect the masses. This reminds me of one of Père's favorite sayings, *"Se rat kay ki manje kay pay."* It is the house rats who eat hay houses. I saw for myself, firsthand, the devouring of these hay houses in the summer of 1997, when I returned to Haiti with a group of students on a trip sponsored by the Ministry of Haitians Living Abroad. Our group was composed of students from France, the United States, and Haiti. This trip was intended to reacquaint people like me with the country that we had left at a young age and connect us with other students our age who were just finishing school in Haiti. While traveling in Haiti with the group, I got to see most of the country. The most startling sight I saw was the number of high-priced Landcruisers and Range Rovers traveling Haiti's roads. I couldn't believe that a country so poor could have people driving such expensive cars. The reason for those cars was revealed to me one rainy day when we were trekking in an old school bus from Port-au-Prince to the southern town of Cayes. I saw young children bathing in the muddy rainwater that had collected in the craters on the road. There were heaps of trash and debris all along the road. Whatever was in this collection of trash must have been decomposing because the smell was unbearable; yet the children washed their little angelic faces, arms, and legs in this sewage. On that day, I finally understood why the rich people need Landcruisers in Haiti: to create craters for the poor to bathe in.

Before that month was over, I got to see Haiti's prosperous sons and daughters at work. We were invited to dinner at Kinam 2, Haiti's Ritz Carlton. The purpose of this assemblage was to network and connect with the rich and powerful so that we could one day return to "rebuild" the country. Over dinner conversations, the students in the group who were living in France and the United States got job offers from the Haitian company heads, but the students living in Haiti were completely neglected and certainly not offered jobs. At that moment, I understood Père's saying about the cigarette burning at both ends and his saying about the house rat eating the hay house.

Pray to the lwas on Saturday, pray to God on Sunday.

In his final letter, Antoine Thurel stated three reasons for which he died: family, country, and religion. Religion is one of the most confusing aspects of being Haitian. Haiti's primary religion is *Vodou*, yet we are even more confused about *Vodou* than the white man who while enslaving us told us it was evil. I once heard a prominent Haitian pastor in Boston say that slavery was God's way of reaching out and saving the African continent. The Haitian parishioners echoed their assent with undiscerning shouts and praises. How long will we continue to pay for this kind salvation? How many Antoine Thurels will die to purge us from it?

I have often imagined Père and Antoine Thurel having a conversation. Père would list his maxims expressing his disillusionment with our people and Antoine Thurel would list his dreams for our outward and inward liberation, the dreams that had motivated him to set himself on fire that morning on August 31, 1987. Perhaps they are having this conversation now in our ancestral African home in Ginen with Boukman, Toussaint, Christophe, and Dessalines; I wish I could hear that conversation. Perhaps I would get some answers to my questions, a few replies that would calm the tormented voices in my head, heal some of my continuing grief over Antoine Thurel's death. Still these questions, like Père's final words, continue to haunt me. Why don't we see that the things we tell ourselves and our children become part of them, and part of us? When will we realize that all of Haiti's children belong to one family, the family of humanity? Why do we teach resignation in our churches? Why do we not respect our ancestors' words and legacy? Why don't we truly honor their sacrifices by treating ourselves and our poorer neighbors more humanely? Will we one day find the answers to those questions, or will we always remain a cigarette burning at both ends?

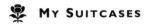 **MY SUITCASES**

Maude Heurtelou

When I was nineteen years old, I left Haiti for Guatemala City to enroll in a bachelor of sciences program. To prepare me for my trip, my parents fixed me two large suitcases filled with farewell gifts: from a bookmark made out of dry banana leaves to family photographs. What I didn't know then is that my suitcases were not only physical but also cultural. These suitcases, both cultural and physical, have been essential to my survival as an immigrant in three different countries.

Upon my arrival in Guatemala City, I whispered my aunt Didine's prayers to the saints, hummed Léon Dimanche's "Nostalgie" while longingly laying out and sifting through the items that had been lovingly packed in my suitcases: the talcum powder on my nightstand, which the vendor at the Iron Market in Port-au-Prince had wanted no payment for because I was leaving for university abroad. The multicolored kite that decorated my wall was made twenty years before by the neighborhood shoeshine man, who had presented it to my mother thinking she was carrying a boy. An unknown artist had sculpted the metal sheet lantern by my window. The small wicker basket in the corner of my room had carried dried Ilan Ilan flowers from my middle school in Port-au-Prince. The embroidered pillowcase where I rested my head each night was made by hand in the mountains of Jacmel. It was embossed with my great-grandmother's initials and passed down from my grandmother, to my mother, and now myself. My rubber sandals, a gift from my friend Marie, reminded me of traveling Haitian feet, steady, firm, and purposeful in their gait. I felt as though the ground beneath me was familiar whenever I wore my sandals. So many things in my suitcases comforted me, while reminding me of home.

Soon my classmates became curious about "*la haitiana*," the one who couldn't speak Spanish at first but was learning so fast. Little by little, I opened my suitcases, both cultural and physical, to them, sharing music, Haitian *konpa,* foods—*griyo,* plantains, rice and beans, *pikliz*—and stories of the feuding Haitian folktale characters Bouki and Malis. One day, I received a surprise visit from the national Guatemalan soccer team. The team was scheduled to compete against the Haitian national soccer team and wanted to look at me to get a sense of what Haitians would look like. Because I was taller than all the Guatemalan players, they assumed that all the Haitians would be very tall as well.

We were the only six Haitians reported to be in Guatemala City: a businessman, a female professor from the French Institute, and three other university students like myself. A few times a year, Claudette, the French professor, would invite me and the other three students to her home. During those afternoons at Claudette's, we would sit on her patio, eat Haitian food, listen to *konpa* music, and share stories from home. The oldest among us, Marijo, came from Jérémie, a southern Haitian town that had produced many famous poets. Marijo would recite verses that described the plush green landscape of the Haitian south. After her poetry recitals, Marijo would walk over to Claudette's piano and play the legendary Haitian ballads, "Haiti

Chérie," and "Choucoune." One other student, Fadia, would dance
while I told riddles.

Krik?

Krak!

You go here. I go there. We meet in the middle. What am I?

A belt!

Those afternoons at Claudette's always eased my longing for
home, if only for a while.

After four years in Guatemala City, I moved to Quebec City, Canada, to look for work, and took my suitcases with me. I carried along
my favorite comb, which I had learned in Haiti could be both a
grooming tool and a musical instrument. To play the comb, all one
had to do was put a strip of paper across the teeth, press one's lips
against the paper, and hum to produce a harmonica-like sound. My
new Canadian friends and I would have evenings of comb recitals
and story telling, turning off the lights for an atmosphere that would
make the stories sound scarier and the comb sound more mysterious.
During cold winter nights, I would entertain my friends with descriptions of the deep earth smell and the thumping sound of Haitian
rain on tin roofs. I would make them ginger root tea and peanut
confections. However there were a few things I resisted sharing. I
didn't tell them that at times what I missed most were the imper-
fections of my country: the large potholes that always forced our feet
or our cars to slow down, the crowds of vendors at the markets who
sometimes made it hard to move freely, but sang melodiously of the
fruits and vegetables they were selling.

One day I accepted the invitation of some friends to accompany
them to the carnival of Quebec. Having been part of the colorful
and lively street party that was a Haitian carnival, I never imagined
that the carnival of Quebec would be an outdoor procession of ice

sculptures in minus-thirty-degree weather. More and more, I began to miss the gorgeous range of colors of Haitian people, from honey, to chocolate, to dark coffee. I missed the aroma of coffee, freshly ground every morning by my neighbors. I missed being greeted with a smile by people who had known me and my family for years. Back home, I had a name and a past, had a family, and a legacy. In Quebec City, I was rootless, just another immigrant.

A few years later, I made yet another move, to the United States, to Florida. At last, I felt, I could rest my suitcases for a while. Florida, home to hundreds of thousands, maybe even a million Haitians, is close to Haiti both in miles and in climate. South Florida, where I live, is full of Caribbean markets whose shelves are stacked with home-grown treasures such as mangoes, plantains, and breadfruits. There are many restaurants, large and small, that serve Haitian dishes like stewed conch and fried goat. Our voices are heard across radio air waves, singing, laughing, and arguing about politics. We have television programs that bring us news and images of home. It is somewhat easier to simulate Haitian life in Florida, but of course being in Florida is not completely like being home.

After more than two decades away from Haiti, I still reach out for my suitcases, both physical and cultural, for all of the items in them, linked as they are to memories and traditions, that have helped me, and still continue to help me survive the immigrant life. However, my suitcase has now expanded with a few more items gathered from other cultures, with the letters and photographs of the friends I have made in Guatemala, Canada, and Florida, with their stories, and languages, and traditions that have slowly merged into my own: the particular lilt of Guatemalan Spanish that I eventually mastered, the hand-made fabrics from San Andrès, the *cabane à sucre* parties in Quebec City, where I indulged in maple syrup candies out on the street, along with the other residents, natives, and immigrants alike.

What my own cultural isolation as an immigrant in these places has taught me is that I am part of a living culture that in no way stops being a part of me, even when I am not completely immersed in it. With everything I do and say, I am perpetuating that culture, enriching it, modifying it when necessary, but contributing to its regeneration. My suitcases, both physical and cultural, have always, and will always, make me proud of my culture. They are perhaps a microcosm of what I am missing living abroad, but will never completely lose.

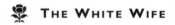

🌹 THE WHITE WIFE

Garry Pierre-Pierre

My wife is white. When I told my friend Rosemonde over lunch that I intended to marry Donna, a petite woman of English, German, and Irish ancestry from Indiana, Rosemonde's jaw dropped as if she'd been hit with a Mike Tyson hook. Rosemonde's reaction foreshadowed what was to come for Donna and me. (We did indeed marry two months later on a cold, rainy December morning in Crawfordsville, Indiana.) If a black friend could have such a visceral reaction, then you know strangers could be far worse. And they have been.

Responses to our being together depend on the level of agitation and gall people have. Most often, we get the *Why is he with her?* stare, the rolled eyes, the sucked teeth. Every once in a while, a brave soul gets cocky, like the sister in the parking lot one day who muttered, "Jungle fever," as we passed by. We paid her no mind.

I know exactly what the stares are all about. Back in my days at Florida A&M University, a crucible of black activism and black power in Tallahassee, I used to be part of that crowd doing the gaping, perplexed and angered by the sight of a black-and-white couple. I took them as an affront to my race. That they happened to have fallen in love was the furthest thing from my mind. Then I fell in love myself, and my old foolishness became what Donna and I have had to learn to deal with. It doesn't faze us now; we've grown immune. But there was a time when we were on constant alert; ignorance is more often subtle—it tends not to shout. Imagine spending every day, walking into every gathering or restaurant, prepared for the slightest insult. It could wear you down if you let it.

Black women and white men seem to be the most offended by the sight of a black man and a white woman. Some black women even seem to feel that my marrying a white woman is downright pathological. I must hate my mother or maybe myself, right? Wrong. I'm not ashamed or sorry or the least bit uncomfortable with my mother, myself, or my marriage. I do, however, get pissed off when my wife is slighted or intimidated, or when she has to contend with ignorant people. When we lived in Fort Lauderdale, Florida, some years ago, a white mechanic helping Donna with a flat tire became furious at the sight of a black-and-white couple driving into the station. "Look at that," he growled as Donna watched him in disbelief. "You would never do that, would you?" Donna opened her locket and showed him a picture. His face flushed red; he blurted out, "But he's educated, right?"

We've come a long way since the days when a black man was lynched simply for making eye contact with a white woman. In fact there are more than three hundred thousand black-white married couples in the United States today, a number that has risen steadily since the 1970s. But still, *this* black man marrying a white woman was a big deal. I was one of those people who once led the arguments against intermarriage. Because racism remains a source of pain for so many of us in this country, many blacks and whites still view interracial couples as unnatural as horses mating with cows. We're treated as if we're traitors in somebody's grand scheme of things. I'm nobody's traitor; I simply followed my heart.

Donna and I met in Togo, West Africa, brought to that obscure place by our mutual idealistic pursuit of trying to make a difference in the world. I was drawn to her midwestern naiveté and easy smile, and she to my northeastern edge and tempo. The attraction—physical and intellectual—was immediate. Even with our differences, we were so much alike. We were both considered radicals in Ronald Reagan's America, where *liberalism* was a dirty word: We had volunteered for the Peace Corps to work in remote rural villages at a time when most of our contemporaries were starting the management training program on the fast track to the Big Time, dreaming of becoming vice president of something. We wanted to teach a trade, share a skill, save a life.

I was born in Haiti and grew up in Elizabeth, New Jersey, a smokestack-filled industrial city about sixteen miles southwest of Manhattan. In the spring of 1987, after graduating from college, I went to Africa to complete the last leg of my own reverse triangular trade. Blacks had left Africa, were taken to South and Central America and the Caribbean, then to the colonies, to keep afloat the peculiar institution that was slavery. I was seeking to connect all the intellectual and spiritual dots. I left FAMU a disciple of Malcolm X (long before X T-shirts were fashionable), and though I never believed in the innate superiority of any race, I was still known to take issue with interracial couples.

So Africa was the last place I expected to be seeing a white woman—the first one I'd ever dated—let alone one I would marry. One of my closest friends, once asked me jokingly, "Garry, did you have to go to Africa to find a white woman? There were plenty in Tallahassee!" I laughed at the irony and thought that ours was in the classic tale of boy meets girl, except boy is caramel-colored and girl is lily-white, and they fall in love in Africa.

When we started dating, I would often ride my motorcycle to

Donna's village in the central part of Togo, a sliver of a country nestled between Ghana and Benin. Over the course of a year, we became closer. I was moved by Donna's spirit and the care and concern she showed when working and playing with the local children. Some nights we would walk into the center of town with a flashlight and the stars as our guide to a watering hole. Between sips of hot beer and bites of fried yams, we wondered aloud about how our lives together would be once we returned to America. Were we getting into something we couldn't handle? I was unsure if I could return to Tallahassee for FAMU's homecoming. I was anxious about the hostility that might come from the all-black environment I remembered. I didn't want people faking it either. But mostly, I didn't want to have all those stunned black faces staring at us, thinking I had let the race down.

After a year, Donna and I started to consider marriage. The thought frightened me. It wasn't because I didn't love her or because she didn't share my journalist's urge to travel and explore. It was because she was white. Being together in African villages was one thing—to them we were simply foreigners—but I would be with a white woman in America. At one point, I thought about calling it off. But then I tried to put myself in Donna's place and wondered how I would feel if she came and told me that she loves me dearly and I would make her a perfect husband, but here was a small problem: I'm black.

We had to deal with our families: We'd told them of our intention to marry, and they knew of our racial difference. Under our intense scrutiny, their welcome was genuine.

Donna grew up in Crawfordsville, Indiana, a tableau of Norman Rockwell's America. She studied psychology at Denison University and had been drawn to Africa since reading a book called *Cherry Ames: Jungle Nurse*, of all things, while in elementary school. Donna's father, Donald Wilkinson, is of Anglo-Saxon stock from rural Illinois. Her mother, Clarissa, is half Irish and half German and grew up in Indianapolis. Neither had ever had much contact with blacks. Still, Donna's mother actually took offense when she learned that her daughter, fearing the worst, had sent her brother a letter before announcing the engagement, trying to gauge their parents' response. The Wilkinsons' welcome was in sharp contrast to the way I was once treated by the mother of a woman I dated in college. Her mother saw me as a cat-eating, *Vodou*-worshipping Haitian American, although I've never tasted the feline and I know as much about *Vodou* as I know about Buddhism. She went so far as to take her daughter, an only child, out of her will in case she lost her mind and married me.

My mother, Yvette, never had any time to harbor ill will toward white people; she was too busy trying to make ends meet and raise me. She, too, embraced the newest member of my family. Getting our parents' blessing turned out to be the easy part.

Some of my friends, like Rosemonde, tried to discourage me from marrying Donna, asking the old question "What about the children?" The race dilemma our kids would face was the least of my concerns: Our world is growing more multicultural by the day, and biracial children are often identified as black. Besides, being Haitian, I've never subscribed to the tragic-mulatto theory. What made the American mulatto's life sad, if it ever was, was not racial identity but rejection by a part of the family. Other relations embraced us as if our union were the most natural thing in the world—as if we were a perfect fit. Donna and I began to see who our friends really were.

As we settled back in the States and headed toward marriage, we confronted more serious problems than racial difference. Several months before our wedding, doctors found a blood clot the size of a golf ball in Donna's head. She underwent surgery to remove it, unsure whether she would ever again be able to speak, walk, or lead a normal life. Then began her recovery: Donna would spend five years on a daily medication and a year in physical therapy, struggling with the simplest sentences. (Today she is healthy but still working to gain full control of her fine motor skills.) Later, as we tried to start a family, she had two miscarriages, one almost took her life.

Other couples may have far less to overcome than we did, but if they're like us, once they decide they're serious, they quickly close ranks against those who would rather see them keep with "their own kind." Nobody's discomfort or anger or annoyance matters more to a couple in love than their being together. We determined that we wouldn't be worn down. Donna and I did this instinctively, without having ever had a conversation about it.

In fact, the first time we talked about how much racism has affected us as a couple was when I started to write this piece. Donna shared her sense of intimidation around some black women, the subtle messages she gets that she's not dressed right or not up to par. "You know when a woman is looking and not approving," she said to me recently, adding that it's something I wouldn't pick up on. "You don't have to have a word said." It angers me that anyone would dare to judge her; she doesn't need to conform to some standard of what a black man's wife ought to be. We also laughed at how some white women take my being with Donna as license to come on to me. A good sense of humor has always kept the ignorant at bay.

It has been more than twelve years since I first met Donna, and after ten years of marriage and two children, we don't have time to worry about what others think of us. With six-year-old Cameron, and two-year-old Mina filling our lives, the stares and whispers of strangers don't matter at all. We have learned to stay away from places where either one of us would be uncomfortable, to choose our friends carefully (we have more black friends than white) and to live in places where we feel safe and secure. That's what any man, of any color, wants for his family.

Since Cameron was born, I've made a herculean effort to make sure that my children are keenly aware of their African heritage. Our walls are festooned with African and Haitian paintings. My music library includes an eclectic collection of jazz, blues, and Haitian and African CDs. This doesn't necessarily mean that my kids won't confront that age-old existential question: Who am I? It is a question that bedevils all of us, regardless of race, religion, culture. I simply want Cameron and Mina to be surrounded by tokens of their African heritage while living in predominantly white America. And we have not shied away from discussing race with Cameron. To him, Daddy is black, Mom is pink, and he is brown. At a recent gathering, when someone pretended not to know this Garry person that Cameron kept talking about, my son simply sighed and answered:

"You know, *black* Garry, my dad."

Everyone laughed.

So if the sight of a black-and-white couple strolling down the street still offends you, it's your problem. We're busy leading our lives and rearing our children and keeping our love alive.

🌹 YOU AND ME AGAINST THE WORLD

Martine Bury

I am sitting in the home of a gorgeous, famous black actor. A hottie. His skin is ebony and his muscles are toned. There are empty beer bottles everywhere, sultry British music playing. And we're at the point in the interview when we get too much like old friends who used to kiss. We reminisce about Brooklyn and the Haitians we knew growing up. He flirts a little. We spill beans about sex and dating. Then he says something and my knees go weak—for I am self-conscious. He says, "You're the kind of sister that would probably turn her nose up at a brother and not give him the time of day." I don't know how he got my number. But I have a story I wish I'd told him in my defense.

I used to be a strong woman. I even considered myself a modern black woman. But six years ago I had to get stronger over eggplant parmesan. I was sitting at a dinner table with the then love of my life and his Texan parents. We were dining at Santerello on the Upper West Side ogling antipasto and getting drunk on red wine. It was a genteel scene. My mother and father were conspicuously absent— visiting with friends somewhere in Queens, where I should have been. My man and I had just announced that we wanted to move to Texas together. I don't know what I was thinking. It was my

Normandy Beach approach to love in full-blown play. So far from East Flatbush where I was born and South Miami where I grew up. Haiti I had buried somewhere just beneath the surface for the night.

These were really reserved Texans, which made the air thick with unanswered questions. We were all laughing in a guarded way. The dining room was claustrophobic in thick red velvets and heavy woods. Still, as I said, I was in love and these were the colors of earth, familiar skin, tall tree trunks, and a dozen red roses. I was wearing a yellow dress to counteract the stress in my face and bring out those undertones people say I glow with. I wanted to be their friendly yellow rose rather than their black rose, in Texan parlance. There's an offensive Waylon Jennings song that goes "The devil made me do it the first time/The second time I done it on my own/ Better leave that black rose alone." Waylon understated, but my boyfriend's mother, under the influence of too much Chianti, would not be stopped. She and her husband began a conversation that went like this. As if I wasn't there:

Mother:	So I just want to tell you that we really like Martine. We think she's great. Ralph and Linda think she's just wonderful.
Father:	Sue!
Mother:	She's smart.
Father:	Sue, shut up!
Mother:	I am just trying to say that we like her but . . .
Father:	Sue. Please.
Mother:	Texas is not New York.
Father:	I'm sorry, Martine. She's had too much to drink.
Mother:	No. Martine. Like I said, we think you're great. What do your parents think about all this?

I ran to the bathroom to cry. Ralph and Linda were their next-door neighbors of Mexican descent who comprised the majority of their ethnic friends. Texas was not New York. Maybe their son and I could live together in New York, or the Bay Area, but not in Texas.

At the time I was not sure just what my parents thought. I never asked because it would have been like talking about sex. In fact, it *would* have been talking about sex. I presumed that in the Caribbean there was unspoken encouragement of interracial dating. Half Indian, part French, two-thirds Arab . . . you know the drill. My father stayed silent on the issue. My mother was agreeable. It was generally the same response they'd had to every decision I ever made. Summer college. Columbia. Brazil. Freelance writing.

I was a student at Columbia University, and I loved the anonymity of New York at nineteen. With a lover you could blend into the throngs, virtually unnoticed. Part of the landscape of the city are the lovers that fit like the fixtures of dilapidated city apartments: original moldings, faucets, and such. Lovers fit in so well against buildings and urban decay because they are so oblivious to the sweat, crowds, and screechy-bumpy arrested traffic. In a Woody Allen movie, you fall in love with falling in love in the city at the Museum of Modern Art or in Central Park. You always notice the lovers, often mismatched, happy to sit too close on packed subways. There is certain freedom in the back of a yellow taxi to stare into goo-goo eyes, touch and kiss, not mindful of the meter, drunk drivers, or a cabby rolling his eyes at the window display of complete lack of self-control. I would sometimes look at the Haitian name on the I.D. card and think, This man could be my uncle or my father.

Before I messed with Texas I'd had my first significant romance with a graduate student in Russian studies. I noticed then the ostracism that would come to define my lovelife. I would hold hands with my boyfriend and members of the Black Students Association would trip on me as I tripped over campus cobblestone and he would stop me from falling. It's hard to say that their stares were hateful or judgmental. Maybe it was just me projecting my guilt for not being the black girl every one wanted me to be. I was, for the moment, maybe the one that the boyfriend wanted. Trying to belong to him, to me, to my family as well as the Black Students Association, the Haitian Students Association, and the Caribbean Students Association (only a few of the groups of which I never officially became a member). It was like Woody Allen quoting Groucho Marx in *Annie Hall* about not joining any club that would have him as a member.

Bedrooms are such sacred spaces because they allow you the freedom to explore the things that are truest about you in dreams and with another body. I couldn't say I saw my reflection in my lover's eyes. But I wondered about his fascination with me. Our skin contrasted as much as our styles did. I had extensions in my hair that he loved to look at—but not to touch. It was hard explaining the hair thing to him when he'd secretly looked as if he wanted to touch something about me that was real. As with my Senegalese twists, the line between real and fantasy somehow was blurred. If I stared at my hand on his stomach long enough it would look like a little brown island on a pale pink sea. I wondered if we could ever disappear into each other. I still think of this rather neutrally. As we do with all private thoughts when we're naked. But outside—if we went too far up the Upper West Side, I would be castigated in a glance or by a declaration. "I can't believe she brought a white boy up in Harlem." As if I wasn't there.

From the time we were eight years old, my best friend from childhood and I would sit around spinning tales and telling each other our dreams. I hate to confess it, but we were expert liars. Still, each day after school we'd report to each other elaborate tales of

how we'd look, what we'd wear when we were twenty and courting
or married to various rock stars and actors. Barring Prince and Michael Jackson, the list was pretty conventional: Leif Garrett, Andy
Gibb, Sting, Rick Springfield, Carey Elwes, and Christopher Atkins.
George Michael and Andrew Ridgely from Wham! took entirely
too big a chunk of our time and creativity. But it went on for years.
Shining white knights who would take us away from our little Caribbean community in Miami. My friend's Jamaican parents and my
Haitian parents were always conspicuously absent from our ritual
imaginings as were families and neighborhoods, patois, *Kreyòl*, *griyo*,
and jerk meats.

By high school we'd grown apart, but we still got together to talk
about relationships—mostly hers. She had a series of sports-playing
significant others. And I'll make it plain: Black boys were not into
me. I tried to be down and alluring. I sometimes even let the basketball and football heroes copy my homework. Romantically, however, it was no go. I read Jamaica Kincaid's *Lucy* my first year in
college. The main character lives in New York and works as an au
pair who sexually crosses racial lines. I got it. It was going to be hard
to be any kind of black intellectual as long as you were sleeping with
the enemy. James Baldwin wrote about this all the time, making the
boudoir the battleground of race war, too.

My grandmother had always shown me photos of my great grandfather who was practically white. She told me while combing my
hair that she had a near ancestor who'd fought in Napoleon's army.
My aunts and uncles and I have always had white friends. Some have
intermarried. I look at my folks' meticulous photo-documentaries of
my birthday parties, which were always exceptionally multicultural.
I know that they didn't orchestrate this universe for me. It's hard
figuring out what my people think of the Man because no one ever
said a word to me until recently.

My hippest aunt and I were munching on sushi once. She reported that there were pretty harsh rumors circulating in the family about the fact that I only date white men. *Only?* was my response. It was the same tone I'd used toward my grandmother when I had my hair braided (and when I went natural). She'd asked me on both occasions: "Do you think you are an African?"

"I am just me," I said, sensing that I was never going to make her happy.

I have to say there is something so surreal about having your lover reach over to you in fascination and ask can he touch your kinky hair or tell you that he has never dated a black woman before. There is something cruel and unforgiving when your lover leaves you because he secretly doesn't know how to take love to the marriage point because of the possibility of beige babies. Or because his family is truly irked by you. And there are a lot of utterly disturbing things men have told me like, "There's nothing hotter than a bald black woman giving me head." (I was not bald!) Or, "I find how dark you are really sexy."

Still, I have trodden very foreign territories. I have had blue lights dimmed and Donna Summer played by boys who listened to Rundgren when disco was the shit because they thought it was appropriate. I was told in bed by a French man that I called to his mind Lauryn Hill—but more *sauvage*. But I have also known sweetness. You know, when it all comes down to warmth and eyes staring into each other. So for all these convoluted reasons, I apologize to the tall lanky writer who loved me so very hard he broke both our hearts. He was so country club that I could not hold his hand on 14th Street because I was freaked out by our juxtaposition. Like many black women with their white boyfriends—I didn't want to draw attention. I averted my glance, especially in Brooklyn.

A couple of years ago my therapist, who happened to be white, asked me why I didn't choose someone else to spill my guts to. Presumptuously, I believed at the time that she was titillated by my dating practices. I probably gave her some song and dance then. It hardly seemed an issue to be tortured by. A boyfriend I accused of fetishizing black women told me point blank: "Some men like blondes!" But there were so many whom I wouldn't really touch or kiss in public because I found it exhausting. I felt similarly about seeing a therapist who looked like me. That I would be outed before one of my own seemed like something terrible. It is hard to understand why I lived in so much conflict. I guess I looked back with my psychologist at a stereotypical history of strong Haitian women who emasculated their men and what-not. But I think it's all bullshit now. I open my bedroom door just a crack to the public. Let the people stare because the people have to see me for who I am. Used to feel like a crumbling fortress with Haitian–Black–American rubble falling fast and fragmenting into a billion little pieces. But no more.

One of the great men of my heart was an entertainment industry bigwig. And I loved his world because I felt free and safe in it. It was my girl-child fantasy. In a larger-than-life kind of life, you can swing whatever way you want because people are gonna give you respect no matter what. Illusory? Yes. But this idea made me stronger.

I used to hate that black male celebs could flaunt their white girlfriends and wives, while you rarely even heard about a black actress's love life. I do thank this man for our romantic dalliance. When he broke my heart, I didn't suddenly become paranoid about the great divide. He had been my closest intellectual and emotional mate. When he left my life, I noticed, like a fool, finally, that pain is just pain. He had once made the most tender observation: He was standing somewhere watching an attractive white man with dreadlocks play with his two *café au lait* babies. He was so enamored with this vision of what he saw as a real option for himself. When we were together, it didn't occur to me that I was an object of conquest or desire. I now open myself to the universe for a true soul companion.

Sure I want a lover who can dance *konpa*, who's read Baldwin and Achebe and Toni Morrison. I want to say something scandalous about what sends my pulse racing, like tan lines and good diction. I cannot say who fits this bill or what he will look like. But at my shrink's suggestion and for my own peace of mind—here is a note to the man I will always love most.

Dear Daddy,

I am told many black women are attracted to men who are the opposite of their fathers. But I don't believe this because I think you and I are so much alike. You are my most treasured model of humanity—loving and complex. No kind of man represents stability or real love better or worse than you do. Just like you, I've always wanted family and community to see me how I want to be seen. So I have unpacked a bit of my emotional baggage. Above are some things about me I want you to learn. I don't doubt that you accept me, I have never worried much about the world doing so. Thank you for letting me be myself.

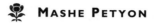

MASHE PETYON

Katia Ulysse

It's been seven years since I have been home. I would run a thousand miles now to reach that man who sits on his little wooden stool, day after day, under the scorching Haitian sun, to sell his art in order to buy more supplies with which to quench the undeniable thirst in his heart. Under the cacophony of shrill voices and riotous laughter at Mashe Petyon, the marketplace at the center of Pétionville, the artist would spend hours watching the vendors and their customers haggling over the price of sugar and bread. Then, with unchallenged genius, he would wave his brushes across the canvas to capture their movements: the fine lines around the women's eyes, the tiny beads of sweat on their brows.

It would thrill me to join those three sun-baked women, barefoot in one of his paintings, as they wash their clothes in a placid brook surrounded by gigantic *mapou* trees and emerald shrubs. I should have been there, at that perfect moment, when the artist painted blue-and-gold water that made concentric circles around and around the women's ankles, the skirts twisted to one side and tucked into waists to stay dry. Only the heartbreaking melodies of Pierre Ciné's acoustic guitar could describe the emotions invoked by the way the scarves are wrapped around the women's heads in hibiscus greens, yellows, and reds.

I would give anything to place my bare hands on the majestic coconut tree that dominates the canvas; its deep green leaves reaching toward the cloudless blue sky, streaked at the horizon with purple, saffron, and amber. At the heart of the shrubs looms the painted shadow of nightfall. Atop it all is a single hut that has one window, one door, and an unseen breeze that gives the thatched roof a permanent sway above which seven black birds hover. Forever.

My friend, who just returned from Haiti, tells me there are few trees left in the mountains; no more lush shrubbery. She says the brooks are parched, leaving rocks buried beneath burning heaps of refuse and mud. The roads are narrow and jagged; many lead to nowhere, and the stench in the streets surrounding Pétionville's cemetery is unbearable.

It's been seven years since I have seen my home. Sometimes when I close my eyes, I envision myself lying on the naked earth inside of my great-grandmother's *peristil*, a modest structure of concrete and clay. The walls of the main room are murals dedicated to ancestors and various *lwas*, the memories of whom must never fade. To the right is Our Lady of Czestochowa; the black virgin has three vertical scars on her cheek. She is holding a child. "That is Ezili," my great-grandmother told me in a hushed voice. "She is the vengeful mother. She will leave you alone as long as you don't bother her child. But touch her child the wrong way, and you will pay." Then my great-grandmother began to sing the same little song I catch myself humming sometimes: "Ezili, they say you eat people. How many have you eaten? Those who speak well, my eyes will protect. Those who speak ill, I will devour."

To the left is a mural of Saint Gerard in his clerical dress. He is standing next to a skull and white lilies on a table. My great-grandmother pointed to that wall and said, "That is Gede." Then she sang a different song: "When they need me, they say I am Gede; when they don't want me, they say I am garbage . . ."

Those melodies will never escape from my memory.

"There are many, many *lwas*," my great-grandmother told me. "Each one has a special song." She taught me the names of all the spirits and sang their songs so that I would pass that knowledge to my own great-grandchildren one day.

Today I live in Washington, D.C., thousands of miles and an ocean away from that *peristil*, from the *lwas*, the spirits, and images that inspired my great-grandmother's songs. But sometimes I find myself on that dirt floor and feel the grains of three hundred years against my skin. I see the rainbow of sequined flags decorating the walls and the center altar, covered with calabash bowls, oil lamps, and layers of candle wax that congealed in labyrinthine patterns. Sun rays filter through the holes in the tin roof, dust spirals heavenward; an avalanche of dreams buries me on that dirt floor, and I am born again.

I see the room that my great-grandmother had forbidden me to enter. I was five years old, holding her big hand, feeling safe among the marred faces of old women out of whose throats ancient chants soared above the flames of bonfires that burned for days to the re-lentless *Kongo* beat of goatskin drums. The elders agreed my eyes were much too young to view the secret room of souls and uncertain crossroads.

The last time I was home I went into that room. My great-grandmother had been dead for years; I felt that I had her permission somehow. The mystery quickly unfolded before my eyes. I had imagined that there would be more substantial things than the altars of cracked cement upon which stood small clay jars covered in layers of orange-colored dust, pieces of deteriorating fabric and broken black and red bead necklaces. The room itself was decaying. Several aluminum plates and containers made from dried calabash shells still bore the traces of disintegrated offerings: corn, sweets, yams and *malanga* just like they sold at Mashe Petyon, a picture of which hangs on my living-room wall.

It has been seven years since I have been home, but I visit Mashe Petyon every morning when I get out of bed with the scarf still tied around my head that keeps my dreams from falling. I look at the wall in my apartment and there they are: an ocean of black women squatting before their wide wicker baskets, their colorful skirts tucked between their legs. These women chatter among themselves, arguing and laughing with sheer abandon.

Sometimes, if the night before was easy, I'm right in there with them laughing as the morning sun travels across the sky, across the straw roof, along my black skin. I rest my head against the wall the way the sugarcane leans against the poles that hold the tent up above the marketplace and keep the invisible lines that divide secure. I know these women who sell bright yellow plastic plates, aluminum skillets, dried codfish, fried plantain, and charcoal. I recognize every one of their faces. Even when the painter exaggerates their features and makes their limbs like giraffes', I get inside the wooden frames and haggle with them the way my great-grandmother did when she took me along to buy the sugar she would sprinkle over sliced tomatoes for breakfast. With a hand cocked on her hip, a serious tone of voice, and steady vigilance in her smoky age-grayed eyes, she would ask for fifty cents' worth of oil, spices, a cup of rice, a pound of beef, and two eggplants to prepare the white-rice-and-legume supper.

It's been a lifetime since I was the little girl-child who sat on the porch at twilight with my great-grandmother, Madan Deo, to listen to her stories about women who shed their skin and took to the skies during the darkest hours of night. Madan Deo told me about the tall man who roamed the streets at midnight and spoke to no one. *Mèt Minwi* was his name, Master of Midnight. I always sat at her knees and faced her so that I would not have to look at the shadows which our little cotton tree threw onto the unpaved road. Shadows and the lamplight often resulted in such a macabre duet.

"*Tim tim?*" she would say before telling me a riddle.

"*Bwa sèch,*" I would answer, giving up quickly because my efforts to solve her riddles would rob me of the chance to hear more of the stories that her own grandmother must have told her. I wish I had asked her why she kept the old dress in which her mother, Madan Zepherin, had died. That dress hung on the wall for many years like a favorite picture.

One night, Madan Deo looked right past me toward the street beyond the porch and said, "*Tim tim?*"

Before I could answer, my great-grandmother stood and walked into the house. She said something about getting a cup of water and that she would return soon. She closed the door behind her to keep the insects from flying inside. Time went by and she did not return. I went to the door and tried to open it. It was locked.

"*Bwa sèch.*" I cried.

I turned to look at the dark road beyond the porch. The long shadow lingering at the foot of the porch told me that someone was there. I pounded on the door and called out to Madan Deo. "*Bwa sèch.* Let me in. I give up. I am afraid."

It has been a lifetime since I was the little girl-child who huddled in the corner of the porch hiding and hoping that *Mèt Minwi* would not see me. I dared not breathe. The shadow waited at the porch. It had a pulse. Someone was there. I dared not look. I wanted to run inside the house, where Madan Deo would keep me safe throughout the night even if a hundred flying, skinless *lougawous* fell through the tin roof.

I opened my eyes for a brief moment. The long shadow stood

still from behind the cotton tree—a few feet from where I was. I covered my eyes again and held my breath.

"Tim tim?" Madan Deo asked.

At last, she had come to save me. I took her hand and tried to pull her into the house. She shook me loose and told me, as she had done many times before, *"Dyab pè dyab; dyab pa manje dyab."* She told me there was nothing in this world to fear. *Devils fear one another but one cannot destroy the other without destroying himself.* I looked into the street and saw the long shadow inching away. It passed before the porch but I did not see him.

"I wanted you to see him," my great-grandmother whispered. "I wanted you to see him the way Madan Zepherin made me see him. Because until you look him in the eye and learn that you can still survive, you will always be afraid of something in this life."

It's been seven years since I walked by the melting black candles and plates of food offerings at the shrine of Baron Lakwa on the way to visit my great-grandmother's grave at Pétionville's cemetery. I thought of the stories Madan Deo recounted about Baron, a *lwa* who stands guard at the crossroads between this life and the other. I thought about the Gede, the spirit that danced in my grandmother's head. They say Gede Nimbo, the protector of children, was her favorite. One of the rooms in the *peristil* was dedicated to him. When I held her hand as a child, during the ceremonies, people often called her Papa Gede. And they would point at me and say, "That child is Gede's granddaughter."

"Devils may fear one another," I can hear Madan Deo say from beyond, "but one cannot destroy the other." And I wonder . . .

Had I not covered my eyes on that warm night so long ago, I would not wake up every morning in search of shadows between the brushstrokes of a painter's version of Mashe Petyon. And perhaps I would not be so afraid to go home today.

❀ POUR WATER ON MY HEAD:
A MEDITATION ON A LIFE OF PAINTING
AND POETRY

Marilene Phipps

GAME OF HEARTS

We all know that to live is to fight. There are two kinds of battles: the ones life demands of us, and the ones we demand of life. Painting and Poetry are my battlefields. And to be honest, I don't know whether they are what I demand of life or what life demands of me: There are days when it is clear that it doesn't make a bit of difference in the world whether I do the work or not—and those days are like rain upon fire—and there are days when it seems clear I have a life mission—and those are wind in the sail.

To me, painting and poetry are living entities, at times unconscious ones, who relate to each other and to me like people in a "relationship"—living parallel lives that occasionally, and hopefully often, intersect intensely and meaningfully, all the while preserving the potential to remain fully independent of each other.

Becoming a painter and a poet had not been a planned, carefully thought-out affair. This persona crystallized after much "meandering." In the years before going to Philadelphia for an MFA at Penn, I had been an undergraduate student in anthropology at Berkeley. It was then that I returned to Haiti and began research in the *Vodou* religion. I wanted to understand the mysterious hushed stories of my childhood. I became initiated.

During this return to Haiti I began to paint. The paintings of that period were probably my first ones to express a kind of exile, a longing for an internal, mythical Haiti—my paradise lost.

WAITING FOR PRAYER

It is clear that all art forms share the same technical concerns, such as form, composition, texture, rhythm, balance. All art forms share the same need to express mood, vision, ideas, and life experience. All art forms require a constant editing so that harmony and tension can work interestingly together. What fuels the creative process are an individual artist's themes, all of which affect the trademark characteristics by which we recognize a work.

Instant recognizable trademark for me: Haiti! I was born in Haiti and growing up Haitian is most of the worth I have. I feel fortunate because Haiti is a place of rich cultural and visual uniqueness. I am a painter from Haiti and I am proud of it. Yet I am sometimes leery of being called a Haitian painter, because this can become a label used to ghettoize.

HAITIAN PASTORALE

I grew up near water, collected tadpoles at a river where women came to wash themselves, their children, their clothes. Men, too, came to wash, and brought their animals to bathe and drink. Water brings life and is used in rituals to evoke spiritual cleansing, renewal, transition to another world:

. . . Pour water on my head
so the sun might glimmer
on me. It is for hope that God
will pull them up by the hair to heaven . . .

Water is part of my vocabulary of exile and of longing. Houses speak of home lost and rebuilt; they shelter the body's memory of life, of dreams, and of God. Doors suggest and allow passages. Windows offer vision, the lure of light, outward or inward.

CARIBBEAN COLLAGE

With my work I try to take people to Haiti—the place where I was born, where I grew up, where my sensibility was formed, my first impressions made. And I take people inside of Haiti, beyond the exotic façade of blue sky, palm trees, beaches, bright colors, and smiling natives; beyond politically disheveled Haiti, economically depressed Haiti, international-aid Haiti, brandishing-sticks-and-machetes Haiti, boat-people Haiti; beyond the America-has-had-enough-of-these-unruly-blacks kind of Haiti. I take people into Haiti's depth, its originality, its richness, its source of strength and creativity, its heart, psyche and soul, its religion, its *Vodou*.

I have often been asked how I can paint such a luminous, exuberant and bright Haiti when all news about Haiti abounds with accounts of the distress of Haitians, and particularly that of the boat people. My response is that I am not an illustrator for *Newsweek*. I am an artist. I don't have to focus on the same events journalists are meant to report. Yes, Haiti is poor and suffers from terrible economic and sociopolitical problems. But that is not all that Haiti is. If either painting or poetry can be seen as a form of prayer, one could say that the brightness in my images is a prayer for Haiti itself. Praying for the color of light is what I am able to do for Haiti with my work as well as challenge the multitude of negative stereotypes the world has been taught about its people.

PRAYER HOUSE

Unique in so many ways, Haiti is the place of another kind of prayer house. Everything in Haiti is permeated by the complex world of *Vodou*. It is the essential filter and fabric of Haitian culture. When I enter the myths and religion of Haiti, I enter a world of exquisite lyrical imagination and freedom, yet of exacting, elaborate, and minutely structured rituals created only to allow timeless wisdom and intelligence to reveal itself to us in spirit possession. *Vodou's* spirits are gathered and ordered within specific families, numbers of which are recognized by and worshipped for their very distinct personality traits and functions.

Living in another country, I use my pen or my brush to voice incantations to a particular world that has created me and, to a certain extent, now uses me to re-create itself.

POUR WATER ON MY HEAD

Technically speaking, I can paint any place, but if I choose one place, it has to do with its meaning—art is an act and effort of communication. Art cannot survive as only a self-indulgent endeavor. Haiti offers me items of meditation into which, because of my particular connection to the country, I can tap and develop further. Cambridge, where I now live, offers me a nurturing environment. Populations of the world are no longer being confined to their original shores. Different cultures are colliding with each other in close quarters and entering each other's consciousness. Through people like me, a Haitian-born painter and poet, foreign imagination is entering the American consciousness and system of reference. Many of us, the uprooted, may have come empty-handed but certainly not empty-hearted. I came with all that I had been and felt before. With all that my parents had been and felt before. With all that my ancestors had been and felt before. With the company of Spirits. So I continue to live and fight even in those days when there is no wind in my sails. I continue to

> . . . Pour water on my head
> so the sun might glimmer
> on me . . .

On all of us.

❦ HALF/FIRST GENERATION

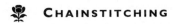

CHAINSTITCHING

Phebus Etienne

After I buried my mother, I would see her often,
standing at the foot of my bed
in a handmade nightgown she trimmed with lace
whenever I was restless with fever or menstrual cramps.
I was not afraid, and if her appearance was a delusion,
it only confirmed my heritage.
Haitians always have relationships with the dead.
Each Sabbath I lit a candle that burned for seven days.
I created an altar on the top shelf of an old television cart.
It was decorated with her Bible, a copy of *The Three Musketeers*,
freesia, delphinium or lilies if they were in season.
My offering of her favorite things didn't conjure
conversations with her spirit as I had hoped.
But there was a dream or two where she was happy,
garnets dangling from her ears,
and one night she shuffled some papers,
which could have been history of my difficult luck
because she said, "We have to do something about this."

She hasn't visited me for months.
I worry that my life is an insult to her memory,
that she looks in and turns away
because I didn't remain a virgin until I married,
because my debts will remain unforgiven.

Lightning tattoos the elms as florists make
corsages to honor living mothers.
I think of going to mass at St. Anne, where she was startled
by the fire of wine when she received her first communion.
But I remember that first Mother's Day without her,
how it pissed me off to watch a seventy-year-old daughter
escort her mom to sip from the chalice.

Yesterday, as the rain fell warm on the azaleas,
I planted creeping phlox on my mother's grave,
urging the miniature flowers to bloom larger next year
like the velvet petals of bougainvillea that covered our
      neighbor's gate.
I crave a yard to plant lemon and mango trees as she did.
Tonight, I mold dumplings for pumpkin stew,
add a dash of vinegar for spice as she taught me,
sprinkle my palms with flour before rolling the dough between
      them.
I will thread my needle and embroider a coconut tree on a
      place mat,
keep stitching her presence in my life.

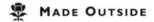

MADE OUTSIDE

Francie Latour

I

It was like a reunion with a stranger. Like many children of immigrants born and raised in the United States, I have skated precariously along the hyphen of my Haitian-American identity. On one side, I bask in the efficiencies of American life: mail-order catalogs, direct-deposit checking, and interoffice envelopes. From the other side, I take the comfort food of Haitian oatmeal and tap into the ongoing debate Haitians love more than any other: politics. It's an endless menu of traits and qualities that I access and draw from, mixing and matching to fit the situation. But I knew that my return to Haiti wouldn't allow me to pick and choose as I pleased. My identity would no longer be defined by me; it would be defined by the Haitians around me.

Eleven years had passed since I had visited the many relatives who still live on the island. I longed to see them and store up new, vivid memories to replace the ones time had turned into faded snapshots.

"Why Haiti?" colleagues in the newsroom asked. Why should a

Hampton Roads newspaper report on a third-world Caribbean island? The question made me impatient.

Why Haiti? Because one year before, Americans had changed the lives of its seven million people by sending twenty-one thousand troops there. Because one year later, Haitians continued to live with—and in spite of—that intervention. And because Haiti's social and cultural landscape is far more textured than the images offered by network television: Haitians as boat people, as AIDS carriers, as *Vodou*-enthralled zombies. There was no excuse for Americans to know so little about, or think so little of, a neighbor whose history and future are so intertwined with theirs.

Still, as I packed my bags, I felt more like an intruder trespassing onto property that was in no way mine, not a proud descendant carrying the torch back to the mainland. What could I tell Americans about a country whose poverty was not my poverty?

My claim to Haitianness was about to be tested. As the airplane touched down on Haiti's cracked soil, the hyphen that held me together started to feel more like the fulcrum of a seesaw whose plank was about to tip on one end or the other.

Haiti, from the window of American Airlines flight 1291, is white sun, blue ocean, brown mountains. Even from this high, the color of the soil is barren and unkind. Since the last time I had this view, much of Haiti's land has been deforested.

Inside, a flight attendant goes into an unusually long explanation about customs forms. She walks through the aisles, where some Haitians flag her down with raised hands. The fact that she is helping them fill out forms they can't read won't come to me until days later.

Outside the airport, the parking lot is a dusty chaos of barbed wire, begging crowds, and obliquely parked cars. The boy begging for money by our car is too young to be a hustler. His fingers hang inside my window; the nails are blunt and crusted with coal-colored dirt. As the car begins to pull away, he doesn't let go. He hangs on and runs with the car, pleading. That is when I make my choice. I stop asking myself how old he is, where his parents are, and when his last meal was. I block him out; I make him disappear. It will be the hardest choice of the entire journey, but it's so easy compared with the life this boy must live.

Beth Bergman, a white American photographer who works for the newspaper, is also here. For Beth, who has never been to Haiti and understands little of its ways, I am an interpreter, a buffer, and a bridge. But to a passerby who eyes us as we make our first forays into the street, I am a traitor. I am the one who has "brought whites to photograph our trash and ask us how much it smells."

To a homeless woman washing off her plate with sewage water, I am an opportunity, for money, for food, for water. Here in this isolated country, where electricity and phone lines are chancy, some of the most media-savvy people I have ever met work their spin of survival on the foreign press.

"I have no money," she says, coming toward us. "I built a house and they tore it down. I have to take my son to the hospital and I can't afford it. What are you going to do for me?"

Without knowing why, I start listing my Haitian credentials: my relatives who live here, my trips here as a child. But this woman is too smart and too poor to care. To her, I am still a stranger. An American stranger.

Beside her, her son, no older than five, looks up into the lens of the camera. Across his face comes the slow realization that he is no longer the same person he was a second ago. He is a commodity now. He's the face of poverty that we will capture and bring back with us to sell newspapers. So he acts accordingly: The liquid brown eyes grow wider, the small hand tugs at mother's skirt, the head tilts with innocence.

I have no right to be surprised at this. As a reporter, I want them to tell me their story; I don't want them to implicate me in it. But how can I fault them? This mother knows already what I am afraid to admit to myself: A one-year anniversary story about Haiti that enlightens Hampton Roads readers won't do anything for her or her baby.

II

It's 7:10 a.m. Sunday. Beth and I stand outside Saint Gerard Church in the cool breeze before the day's punishing heat sets in. It took hours to pick out the one nice blouse I knew I would need to bring for church. Dressing up is part of Sunday worship, no matter how rich or how poor one is. Etched in my mind are black-and-white images of my mother as a young girl in a ruffled white dress bordered with lace, her cotton socks perfectly folded over.

Today, women file in through the church doors in long, cotton dresses and checkered skirts; the men wear paisley ties and leather shoes.

Just before I take my seat inside, a woman next to me points to my sleeveless silk shirt and whispers, "They're not going to give you communion dressed like that. You didn't cover your arms enough. You need sleeves."

But later as we wound our way of the capital's main cemetery, where Catholic rites merge with *Vodou* rituals in sacred beauty, I realize that I would need far more than a pair of sleeves to belong.

III

For many Haitian immigrants and their children, *Vodou* is a loaded word. Nine years ago, I watched an episode of *Miami Vice* through what I thought were Haitian eyes. I hated it. In my mind, it invoked pretty much every stereotype of *Vodou* and the Haitians who practice it. By the third commercial break, *Vodou* serum had turned Detective Tubbs into a zombie. Dazed by the pounding chants of crazed Haitian worshippers, the rogue cop became possessed. He twitched miserably with fever. Even his partner, Crockett, couldn't snap him out of it. From the TV in the basement of my parents' house, I smoldered in anger. No one watching this would understand the complexity of this African-based religion that meant so much to Haitians, nor the symbolism of the gods that made up its hierarchy.

At the entrance to the main cemetery in Port-au-Prince, a sign in black letters reads, YOU ARE NOTHING BUT DUST. On any given day here, solemn processions of mourners draped in rosaries prop each other up as they walk beside caskets. But today, what we find is an angry woman determined to curse an enemy.

It's the first *Vodou* ceremony I've ever seen, and I can't make sense of it. The woman splashes clear moonshine and dark rum around a charred stone cross. On a straw chair in front of the cross, a flame burns inside a metal bowl. Her thin, tough arms tie a rope around the cross into a tight knot. Later, she will toss salt and crack eggs around the cross to ward off any bad spirits that could interfere with her mission.

"She's calling on the god Baron," Faubert, our driver, tells me. "Baron is a *Vodou* god. When she ties the rope around the cross, it's like she's tying it around a person. And from now on, when that person tries to do anything, he won't do it right. He can do nothing good anymore because Baron has that person tied up."

Beside me, Beth is crouched down, snapping pictures. I hear the opening and closing of the shutter in slow motion, and my thoughts split off in all directions. How is what comes through my lens any different than the view from Hollywood cameras that once enraged me? I try to unravel the symbols and chants, but I keep hitting a cultural wall. I don't have the knowledge.

I V

In the warped recesses of my mind, I ask myself this question: If I were ever put on trial by a Committee for Haitian Authenticity, how would I defend myself? How would I explain what has led me and my friend to this place, scribbling and shooting furiously for an American audience?

At the end of my workday, a battery of questions awaited me at my grandmother's house in Pétionville, a suburb of Port-au-Prince. Was I doing well in my career? How is my older brother, her godson? Did I have a boyfriend? Would I ever bear her great-grandchildren? And why did I cut my hair so short?

"You've accomplished too much in your young life to be walking around with a head like that," she says, inspecting my closely cropped cut. "You've got to think about getting married."

When I used to come to Haiti with my family, this is where we would stay. Each step through the house brings back another mem-ory: the blue-green bathroom tiles where I nursed mosquito bites with Caladryl and cotton swabs; the kitchen where my grandmother stirred long sticks of cinnamon and vanilla extract into the breakfast oatmeal; my uncle Eddie's room off in the corner where no one was ever supposed to go.

Standing over the dining-room table, she shows us pictures of her cruise on the *Queen Elizabeth II* and her journeys in the Spanish countryside. "I am eighty years old," she says, "and I have lived a good life." That is all she wants for her children and her grandchildren.

V

When I graduated from college three years ago, my grandmother came for the long day of ceremonies. When they called my name to receive my diploma, my grandmother shouted louder than anyone else. I could actually hear her cheering as I climbed the steps and reached for my degree. I am the granddaughter who has succeeded in America.

"You were made outside." This is the way many Haitians speak of those of us who were born or grew up in the United States. It is as much a badge of pride as it is a stinging resentment. The ones made outside have proven how well Haitians can flourish in the land of opportunity. But, in all our successes, we have also abandoned them. For Haitians who have struggled through the poverty and terror of daily life, there is no room for hyphens in a person's identity. Because I have not suffered with them, I can never be of them. The best I could hope for was to make my journey count. To take everything I was told and shown and tell a story in which both Haitians and Americans could see a sliver of themselves and of each other. A story that didn't tell the truth, but told the many truths I could never tell alone.

🌸 THE MILLION MAN MARCH

Anthony Calypso

It was about 10:30 p.m. or a little bit later when I started walking down the hill to the convenience store at the Mobil Station on Broadway. I couldn't figure out what snacks to buy for the trip because I didn't get to take trips very often. I can count on one hand how many times I've left town.

I took the long way down the hill, and ran into a friend of mine from Albany who was already two hours into his journey by the time he'd made it to Nyack.

"You going to the March?" he asked me. This brother had these big eyes and as I peered into his car in the darkness, they looked like floodlights. I felt something beginning to pump in me. I wanted to hop in the car with him and start the road trip right then and there, but I had a ticket for the bus, and about an hour longer to wait before it left. I looked again at his eyes and we started talking the way brothers talk sometimes. It's in the eyes. Like, say the both of us were checking out the same girl. The eyes might say, "Did you catch that?" Or if I was looking at some other cat's girl, the brother might stare me down or UPS me a quick message with his eyes like, "Bro, she's with me. You can stare up and down, but ain't nothin' you can do about it—might hurt your eyes, too." It's all in the eyes sometimes.

Anyway, I told him to watch out—there was going to be a massive police force all over the highways on the route to D.C. I hoped to convey this warning to him with my eyes, "It's October fifteenth, brother. Be careful on the road. Everyone knows about the March." There was way too much electricity in the air between us to even mouth that.

It finally started to click that I, too, was headed to the Million Man March in Washington, D.C. The March was all over the news. I had caught a clip on CNN of some brothers who were from Seattle; they were already there. When I saw my boy jet off with a carload of folks to D.C., I felt like I was late even though the march hadn't really started yet. There was a current running through my body, pulling me like a chain. *Get to D.C.*

The street felt quiet, as if something was going to happen, that this something was so massive that a path would have to be cleared in order to move through it—I left the Mobil with a couple of snacks—some pudding, chips, a Snapple. I had a turkey sandwich at home. On the way back to my house, I ran into this cat who I only knew by sight.

"You know where we were lining up?"

"Corner of Franklin and Depew."

I walked with him around the corner and back to Franklin Street. I lived one block up from Franklin. As we walked up the street together, he started telling me about how he'd said good-bye to his folks. He asked me if I had said good-bye to my folks yet.

"Good-bye?"

"Yeah, man. I told my moms and all my folks that if I don't make it back from D.C.—if something happens to me down there—I told them that I loved them."

"Word?"

"You gotta say good-bye to them."

Until he'd said that, I'd had every intention of making it back from D.C.—I hadn't thought about just how much could go wrong down there.

We were on Franklin talking and I was going to see him again pretty soon on Franklin. And the thing about Franklin—or at least the part of it where the bus was going to pull up—is that it's undeniably black. It's a pretty safe bet that if you walk or drive down Franklin, something in the air will give you the sense that it's a black neighborhood. It may be a couple of cars parked on the street corner playing music. Or a small crew of fellas talking on the corner, shooting dice, or just hanging out next to the laundromat. Or it may just be an unmarked police car circling the block. You might find some older folks sitting on porches, too. There are loud conversations here, and a person passing by might get to hear the way black folks can transform English. It can sound dirty, but crisp and proper too, on Franklin, and whichever way the language comes out, it seems somehow to lurk along the street. When kids play or yell down this way, it feels like their voices stick to the metal bars that surround the projects. In the same way, when the older folks talk, their words drift into the wall and live deep inside the brick and cement. A good chunk of black culture resonates at this intersection of Franklin and Depew. And because of that, this particular intersection makes the rest of the town look lily white.

Franklin is the first street you hit coming from the city, and it stretches from one side of town to just about the end of it—it goes from the rich to the poor sections, and it holds truth, with blood and footsteps smeared all over it. Footsteps can go any direction on Franklin Street. Space is tight here at this intersection. Everything here happens right on top of everything else. The projects form an imaginary border on Franklin Street, and they are surrounded by parking lots. The only vacant piece of land has been fenced off and transformed into a community garden. It's the only lush, green place in the area. At any given moment during the spring and summer, you'll find people in the garden nursing the vegetation. They have come to Franklin to do that.

I lived just off the intersection of Franklin and Cedar Hill when I was little. A couple of Rolls-Royces were always parked across the street in front of a garage. They were a customary part of the view from my living-room window. When I was a kid, I was poor and happy. As I got older, I began to feel poor and desperately hurt somehow by that feeling. I began to see differences, I began to feel what being poor was really about; and there was a constant blur in my vision because of that feeling. It made everything else feel blurry. The feeling gnawed at me, and for a long time being poor was the only detail I could actually focus on. I could almost hear it ringing in my head all day long. "I'm poor." It all looked poor. Everything. Every day I thought about it. I thought about the grime and the roaches and I thought about being called Haitian like that was a bad word. There is a woman who I still see now and then on Franklin Street. When I was little, she used to bang on our windows and scream, "Haitians, go home!"

There is very little distance between Franklin Street and myself. I grew up having to pass along Franklin every day, and however the street felt, it affected me. If it felt Haitian, then I did too. If it felt American, then it became a problem for me because I was an American who felt like a Haitian. If the street was quiet, then somehow I felt a little quiet also. Franklin Street was dead the day the rapper Scott La Rock was shot. Nothing happened. Nothing moved. I remember that much.

But the cat I was talking to right there on Franklin, and myself, any other cat who has crossed through Franklin, laughed on Franklin, fought on Franklin, or cried on Franklin; and anyone who has spent a hot summer night on Franklin trying to keep cool—about being poor or about being—makes up a part of this street. And anyone who has feared Franklin or felt the white on Franklin, or anyone who has felt Haitian on Franklin or anyone who has felt strong because of Franklin has meshed with the voices of this street and become part of it. And for whatever subtle, American reason, the bus to the Million Man March was going to pull up right on the corner where, if you want, you can get a forty-ounce bottle of malt liquor or a three-dollar bottle of scented Muslin oil.

The electricity had me rattling off to my aunt when I got home from the Mobil. I had an uncle there too; he was visiting from Haiti and this was his first trip to America. He wanted to go to the March and I had been scrambling to try and find him a ticket for the bus. I even tried to get him a ride with the first brother I met on Broadway who I knew I could trust. My uncle didn't speak any English, so I couldn't send him down with just anyone. So when my boy told me that he wouldn't have room, I felt like that was it, there wasn't any way to get him to D.C. Maybe if there was space on the bus I could buy him a ticket at the lineup. I asked him if he was willing to go to the lineup, but by then the idea of going to the March was over for him.

"*Lese sa,*" (Forget it, no big deal) he said to me.

When I got home, I crisscrossed the apartment trying to get everything together. I had maybe a half hour before the lineup. The battery to one of my cameras was still charging when I picked up the phone to call my mother. It was one of those calls I didn't want to make because the woman panics even when I go into the city for the day. She told me to be careful and underneath her voice I could hear her deepest thoughts. *Boy, I wish you wouldn't go. This doesn't even concern you. Your entire family is Haitian. The March is for Americans. You're not an American, not entirely. Why do you always have to be the activist? What are you going to the March for?* I didn't tell her that I loved her because I couldn't bring myself to believe I wouldn't be back and that this phone call was the last time I would speak to her.

But in the far outer left corner of my mind, I pictured a sudden unexplainable gas pipe explosion occurring on October 16, under D.C., in which a million plus black men die—story at eleven. With that idea in my head somewhere, I took my bus ticket out of its envelope. I had bought it the week before the March and every day when I came back from class I'd check the envelope because I'm neurotic. I needed to see that it was where I had left it. The first time I brought it home I snapped a picture of it and then put it in a drawer underneath some folders. My heart would start to race if I didn't see it immediately when I opened the drawer. Every day the envelope slipped underneath more folders. By the end of the week I checked it a couple of times a day. It looked like an invitation that someone might get for a graduation party. The ticket had put an end to about a year and a half of just talk. I said good-byes to my aunt and uncle and walked down the hill.

There were two brothers standing on the corner. The street was still a little quiet. I had the time and the space to try and set up a shot of the two guys, so I stepped out in the street and took the picture. A red jeep pulled up and then all of a sudden a caravan of cars pulled up to the curb. There was a mass of black people standing on Franklin, which is to say that aside from the actual physical bodies on the street there was also in the night a monstrous spiritual presence almost shaking the ground the way the floor shakes during a fraternal step show. It felt that spiritual—like somewhere above us there were slaves floating by and maybe there were some porters in the area with some railroad workers. There had to have been a few souls watching us on Franklin, maybe even the spirits of those who drowned in the sea on the way over here. I would love to believe that there was a whole congregation up there watching us and elbowing themselves in a frenzy, thinking themselves that this was what they waited four hundred years to see.

There were footsteps everywhere, and all sorts of brothers about to board the bus. There were women waiting too. They had come to send off their mates and husbands, their fathers and their sons. The scene was a little chaotic now, but at the same time it was very calm. The hustling and bustling on the corner of Franklin felt great. No one got angry and several fire engines crisscrossed the intersection where the bus was about to pull up—it was odd to see them driving by, particularly since an alarm hadn't gone off at all that night.

I started snapping pictures randomly. I took a shot of a woman looking out into the street; she was clutching her daughter from behind. The little girl smiled for me. Her tiny face and her half-shut eyes spill out from underneath the hat she's wearing. The mother looks pensive, she doesn't even notice the camera. The look on her face reminds me of how worried my own mother must have looked when she spoke to me on the phone.

A large gray bus rumbled over to the corner, and the line moved across the street to where the bus pulled up. A brother with a bow tie, a representative from the Nation of Islam, walked by real quiet and it felt like everyone's eyes were watching him and waiting for his instructions. He was going to ride on the bus with us to D.C.

The noise died down. We were told that we should have our bags opened so they could be searched. The search was about not taking chances. We could get stopped by the police at any point on the road for whatever reason. It was a light search, a happy search— I've been searched by the police before, and it feels much different. I was searched by the police for less than twenty seconds, but as I put my hands on the hood of the car that night, I had this swelling underneath the muscles in my eyes because it was clear there was nothing I could do about the search and about always feeling like I was under suspicion just for being a young black male. That night I was with a couple of friends and the police pulled us over for not having our headlights on. I can't say what I was thinking, but as the white policeman approached the car I had stepped out. It was a silly mistake, because as soon as I stepped out of the car, I became suspicious to him and he frisked me. I must admit, to the officer's credit, he was incredibly professional. I guess I just wanted him to see me as an individual, not as a suspect. Another time, I was walking down Broadway to get a cup of coffee; I watched a police officer follow me in his squad car all the way up the street. Finally he pulled over and asked me for identification. "You look like someone I might be looking for," he said. I have never committed a crime. But I showed the officer my I.D. that American night.

By now it was a liquid black night and if the ticket could talk it would have said that my fingers felt like bricks against its skin because I clutched onto it until the time came to fork it over. I got on the bus and moved toward the middle. Years ago I thought the back of the bus was the only place I could sit. It was where the cool people sat. It was from these folks that I learned a thing or two about having dark skin and about having nappy hair. These were all the things that belonged somewhere in the back. They were supposed to be underneath, hidden away in a trunk in some closet. They felt connected somehow, and they never left my mind even when I was trying to be cool—and being cool was the most important thing for me back then. Being cool meant that I was accepted. Among these people, all of whom were pretty much marginalized by poverty, I had another layer of blackness. I was one of these Haitians—those boat people, those funny-clothes-wearing people, those cats with

AIDS, those people who speak funny. My uncle, not the one who asked to go to the March with me, had to fight his way back and forth to school when he first came to America from Haiti. Once, another uncle told me that I was from Africa. I didn't buy it for a second. When I was about nine, I developed an answer if someone asked if I was Haitian: I would say that I was West Indian. I was born here, and had never stepped out of this country, but no one accepted me as an American.

My favorite subject in grade school was history—I loved Washington, I loved Jefferson, I loved the war cards that Time/Life used to sell because they had stories on the back of them. I loved the American Revolution. I didn't love Crispus Attucks, a black hero of the American revolution, the first man killed in the Boston Massacre. I didn't know who he was. I loved the War of 1812. And in a school chock full of Haitian-American kids, we didn't learn a thing about the Haitian trinity of revolutionaries Jean-Jacques Dessalines, Toussaint Louverture, and Henri Christophe. It was only after getting out of the school system that I learned about American blacks and about myself. I was angry then, because when I finally began to get a sense of who I was and what I wanted to become, I regretted all the time I had wasted believing what other histories and other institutions said about me.

The bus got quiet for a couple of minutes before we rolled off. The elder cat on the bus led a prayer—we asked God for a safe trip. A couple of seats away there was a father sitting with his son, and I studied them hard. A part of me always studies a father sitting with his son. It's an involuntary act. As I watched them talking back and forth, my mind slipped back to another time when I was on the phone with a friend of mine. I made a joke and he started laughing and in the background his father started laughing too. The sound of the two of them laughing in clumsy union kept playing in my head.

It became like music to me, listening to them laugh. Those notes of a father and son's laughter blended with the voices of the father and son next to me on the bus. The sound conveys a certain feeling to me. It's a certain sound that I have never had with my own father. When I heard my friend on the phone with his dad laughing, I realized there was a key sound that was missing whenever I shared a laugh with my father. Every laugh I've ever had with my father has been guarded. It's always been a weary laugh with him. There has never been just an easy, natural laugh between us. When I laugh with him on the phone or when I'm sitting in front of him, there's always something triggered, something underneath, and it always cancels out any comfort or ease that we might have felt. Every laugh has always been like two strangers breaking the ice, but over and over again. When I heard my friend on the phone with his father and when I saw the father and son on the bus together, I was overwhelmed by a sense that this laughter happened for these fathers and sons on a regular basis.

The men on the bus were like an extended family. Some of them I already knew; some had lived on or around Franklin. The word *brother* was used over and over. We were all brothers at this point, bound together by the same goal. The buzz on the bus felt a tiny bit divine. The last thing I remember before dozing off was the cool and steady purring of the bus engine. A brother was at the wheel and a brother owned the bus.

I woke up once to hear the bus driver arguing with a truck driver over the CB. The trucker had a southern drawl. He had said over the air, "I hear a whole bunch of niggers are heading down to D.C." It didn't sound real. I woke up to hear this drawl over the driver's CB and in that drawl I heard some of the reason I was going to the March. The casual and deceptive way that the trucker used the word *nigger* over the airwaves really got to me. It wasn't so much him, but more the general feeling that what he was saying was accepted in a broad American sense. It was that attitude I was hoping to counter by going to the March. I did not want to end up just as another American statistic. I did not want to show up in some American catalog as another young black male dead or in prison. I did not want to be beaten or disgraced by a cop who felt that it was okay to brutalize or kill a black male based on an accepted American suspicion of him, which on any given day, could mean me. On any given day my mother could get the call. Mrs. Calypso? We found your son with a gun. (I've never carried a gun or any weapon). Ma'am, your son looked suspicious. (I wear my hair in long dreadlocks.) We questioned him. He resisted the arresting officer. Please come and identify the body.

I wanted America to know that if my only crime was being black, then my mother would never survive that call. I wanted America to know that no mother can survive that call, and that call destroys families every day. I wanted America to know that there are families all over America trying to pick up the pieces that some Lone Ranger left behind while on his shift. I wanted America to know that I just want to work and live without any interruption of that. I wanted America to feel Franklin Street. I wanted America to know that I had been at a job for close to seven years and a white male on the job less than six months made more than I did. I wanted America to try to understand the kind of humiliation I went through every time I went to the bank to cash my check. There was more. There was much more.

By daylight we were in D.C. Radio reports stated that at least half a million other black men were pouring into the place at that very moment. Women waved to us on their way to work. They had a gleam in their eyes and I'm sure I did too. Part of the March was about this; it was about reconciling with women. And for me, it was just the first step. Maybe this would help me laugh—just laugh a good clean laugh. We got off the bus and walked toward the subway.

The train ride had everybody laughing somehow because the cars were packed—I don't think our car could have held another body. There was a young white woman on the platform who stood right next to me. In front of all these black faces, her own color must have gone through her mind, but I didn't get the feeling that she felt threatened. I spent the rest of the day obsessed with observing white people who were at the March. I would watch them and try to snap their picture.

As we emerged from the train, two Muslim women watched us from a trailer window. They never looked at me. One woman in particular had beautiful, piercing eyes. Our group dispersed into a sea of black men. By eight o'clock in the morning it was impossible to get to the front of the Washington Mall. I could not fathom the number of people I saw whenever I looked back into the crowd. Every tree was occupied; every statue framed with bodies; there were even people perched on stoplights. I was drawn to a group of Rastafarians who had formed a circle and were playing drums. I moved around with my uncle the entire day. We just kept moving as we met brothers from everywhere. I met a woman from the Bahamas. I looked up to one of the massive monitors to see who was speaking. The man said he'd just received a fax from Africa, and they were watching us. There was thunderous applause. Sometime later Rosa Parks stepped up to the microphone. I was awed to think that this tiny, delicate woman had helped bring us to the mall by refusing to sit in the back of a southern bus and starting the Civil Rights Movement. Without her, the March might have never existed. I saw her on the monitor and it was the first of many times that day I wanted to start crying. Her frail voice rang in my ears. I could feel my eyes getting really moist and I fought to keep from crying.

I fought that feeling all day. As a race of men, I felt like we had never really arrived until that day. The March was a step toward being seen as human. It felt like redemption to me. At no time did I feel nervous. Even if a bomb went off in the middle of the crowd, it felt like the spiritual presence of all our souls and those watching from above could and would contain it. And maybe the absence of that paranoia was what made me feel like crying. I didn't cry though. I had been holding back the water of my eyes long before the March. I still have the water from the March and water from before. I still have these tears. I have new ones, too.

I went off to one side and was about to sit down when I saw a white man standing like a pillar in the ground. He was frozen. He was holding an American flag upside down and he held a cardboard sign in front of the flag. The sign read: A MILLION AND ME. Scrawled on the flag were the words: UNITED WE STAND DIVIDED WE FALL. The man had large, ice-blue eyes and somehow he looked cornered. I didn't want to get too close because I was unsure just what he would do. He looked like a real-life Marlboro man. I guess I was scared of this man's courage, too. If someone called for a million white men to come to Washington, D.C., I would never show up, and I have good reason not to. At first, I figured this guy was some zany, white-boy leftist. I walked away from him, but I kept thinking about him. It took a couple of years and an incidental conversation before I realized what message he was conveying with the flag. In the military an upside-down flag is a distress signal. The truth of it shook me hard. There could never be an all-white or an all-black concern, we can't escape each other that way.

As we were leaving the mall and heading back toward the bus, Minister Louis Farrakhan of the Nation of Islam began speaking. I only caught bits and pieces of his speech as I made my way through the streets of D.C. His voice floated through the air, his tone dipped into a subtle call, and he paused elegantly, then shifted as his speech became more serious. He spoke about responsibility, and the word hammered over the P.A. system and it sank into my eardrums and that was the message I carried home with me. I heard it over and over as I left the mall. Thousands of people registered to vote at the March, hundreds of thousands latched onto ideas and a million plus probably felt reborn or at least rejuvenated somehow. For me the March happened in tiny clips. Every step I had taken led me to D.C., and what America was moving toward and how it changed and how it stayed the same led me to D.C.

Most of the group from my neighborhood in Rockland County walked back together to where the bus was parked. Minister Far-rakhan could be heard for what seemed like miles around. We boarded the bus and he was still talking. The sign on the bus read: THE CHICKENBONE EXPRESS. Someone next to me remarked that he was offended by the stereotypical implications of the sign, that all black people love chicken. The sign didn't bother me at all; what had happened on the mall that day had stomped all over any stereo-type someone might have wanted to use. To me, the sign was harm-less. Besides, I love chicken and I'm black. Pass me some chicken, I'll deal with the stereotype in my own way. *Gracias.*

I was going home reconciled. I felt American. I felt I had taken part in an American tradition. I felt our numbers couldn't be ignored and I felt that a lot of discussion that day all over the country would have to include black males and it would have to include a different way of looking at us. I didn't go home "angry" at anyone. In fact I felt better about America as a whole. I sensed from all the eyes around me that something very deep had been resolved for a lot of brothers. There hadn't been any violence to disrupt the March. And we were alive. There was no bomb under D.C.

I saw a brother the next day walking with his son on Franklin. I had never seen him walking with his son before. He had been on the bus. I made my way to the deli where I usually eat lunch and got into a conversation with a family from Tennessee. It was probably that drawl of theirs that provoked me into conversation with them. I had been talking about the March to someone else and the older southern woman looked at me and said with an intriguing twang that she had been "praying for us." I believed her. I believed what her eyes were saying to me, and I thanked her for her prayers because her prayers had fused with the spirit I was carrying from the March. I believed her because I imagined that everyone had been watching and praying for us. The slaves had been watching. The Quakers had been watching, and so had John Brown, Nat Turner, and George Jackson. Jean-Jacques Dessalines, Toussaint Louverture and Henri Christophe were watching. So was Crispus Attucks. Servicemen like him were watching from their posts. And heroes were watching from their graves. The white man with the distress signal was watching somewhere. I believed her drawl. I believed her eyes. And for that moment, it felt impossible to be invisible.

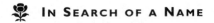

✿ IN SEARCH OF A NAME

Miriam Neptune

1980

My first nightmare was provoked by a doll. She sat on my toybox, regal in her peasant dress and scarf. I dreamt that she cackled, and attacked my *Spiderman* comic book, then went after me. My mother saved me. She took the doll away and sent it back to my father.

I imagined my father as a bogeyman, like the *macoutes* my mother described to me from her childhood—they would take you away in the night. My father would arrive unannounced, with the court order, to take me for the weekend, even if I kicked and screamed, even if my mother cried.

1986

In the fourth grade, we presented our family stories to the class. I announced that my parents were from Haiti. I repeated what my mother had taught me in singsong tones, "Haiti shares an island with the Dominican Republic. It is next to Puerto Rico and Cuba." My classmates laughed. They had already decided that I was an alien.

The only Haiti they could imagine was an island where "everybody *hates* each other."

1986 was the year my father left. I remember he drove by our house in Los Angeles on his way to New York with his new family. He sent for me during Easter. I remember not caring. Maybe a father was like a first cousin—someone you played with once a year.

On one trip my father and I explored the city together, recording everything we saw. There is still a magic that takes over when I remember holding his camera for the first time. As we stood on the edge of Central Park, I narrated, "Here we are in New York City, across from the Natural History Museum, and Central Park. Let's see how many interesting things there are. There are dogs, there are bus-waiters, and fathers." As I zoomed in on his face, he cautioned, "I think you are little bit too close."

1986 was also a big year for Haiti. Mommy and I watched as Baby Doc and his wife fled with the national treasury in a silver Mercedes. Baby Doc really was a big baby—a boy, whose father made him president at nineteen, who ran away when his toy soldiers began to burn.

I finally thought to ask my mother how long it had been since she was home. "Twenty years," she replied. I could not imagine time that long.

1989

When I turned thirteen, I was finally allowed to watch *The Serpent and the Rainbow*, the horror movie everyone had seen but me. I remember feeling captivated by Marielle, the young Haitian doctor who guides an American on his journey to find the "zombie drug."

I was taken in by her elegance, her ability to move so fluidly between this world and the beyond. She was a dancer, the embodiment of Erzulie Freda. This was the type of Haitian woman I wanted to be.

My dream ended when I viewed her making "love" to the American, scratching at him gently like a lioness eating her pray. I understand now that Marielle is just another black exotic, and the story is not about her. I searched for other images. What I found was the Haiti of an American imagination, an island of a million horrors. Haitians were zombies, mobsters, and angry witches. The movies I found failed to depict the true horror: that we were a prideful people being eaten by the shadow of colonialism, unable to speak for ourselves.

1991

At fifteen, I started to care more about Haitian politics. I read everything I could about Aristide. He was like my Nelson Mandela. I saw him as the only hope for democracy in Haiti. I watched as he rose from champion of the poor to president of the nation, then was plucked from his pedestal and muzzled like a rabid dog. I learned not to put all of my eggs in one basket.

On my fifteenth birthday, my father reappeared. He brought me more rice and beans and cake than I could eat. He told me the story of how he met my mother at a wedding in Brooklyn—she was wearing an orange dress.

We took a picture together, and for the first time I realized our smiles were the same. My mother accused me of betrayal. "Your father's family are Duvalierists," she said, warning me that he could not be trusted.

1994

In the middle of the coup, my mother taught me to speak out about the way we were treated. She put me on stage one night a meeting of peace activists, and told me to describe what I knew about the raping and killing of dissenters in Haiti. My voice cracked and my knees shook as I felt her pass on the burden to me, to represent us.

I thought of taking my mother's name, Bateau. Boat. I imagine the boat, floating on the seas with no place to land. How could I take that name when even she chooses not to associate with the father who gave it to her?

1995

Twenty years have passed, and now it is my turn to go home. As I board the plane to Port-au-Prince, I am suddenly conscious of my bent shoulders and drab clothing. The woman ahead of me in a bright blue dress holds her head high, despite the weight of the sacks she grips in each hand. If someone at this moment were to ask me who I am, I would not know how to respond.

When we arrive, a small band plays ballads on the runway. The man checking my passport stares at me then decides to speak English instead of *Kreyòl*. I am an election observer, an American who brings some semblance of justice by recording the voting process. We hover over college students as they count ballots at midnight in Les Cayes. We count them again, and write down our results. The answer is easy: René Préval has won. Twenty percent of voters have voiced their opinion. The other eighty percent watch silently as "democracy" changes hands.

The morning after the elections in Les Cayes, a man approaches me to ask my name. I tell him, "Miriam Neptune." He says I am his second cousin, the daughter of his first cousin. The Neptunes live here, he tells me. I smile at the coincidence, but cry inside because the name is only a name, not a family.

1998

Does name determine lineage? The only lineage I embrace is the one that raised me: my mother, her mother, and the mothers who created her. What is nation? What is my nation? Nation is in part, the imagination. Nation exists only where we create boundaries. My nation lives in the waters between spiritual and physical homes.

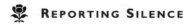

🌺 REPORTING SILENCE

Leslie Casimir

I make a living by telling other people's stories. These people are all strangers to me, a newspaper reporter, yet I am often able to convince them to pour out some of their most intimate thoughts, dreams, and miseries—details that are usually shared between close relatives, passed on from grandmother to granddaughter, mother to daughter, father to son. I can look grieving women in their watery eyes and ask them to describe their murdered sons or husbands—their ambitions, their scent. And amazingly enough, they will comply. I am moved to tell their stories for I am not certain of my own.

Details about my family have avoided me all of my life. In my twenty-nine years, I have been trained not to expect to learn much about the women and men who came before me. They are dead, my only surviving grandmother often insists. What would be the point in raising the dead? *Leve mò.* This is an expression I have heard over and over again. An expression I have grown to accept. A phrase that angers me. Frustration from not knowing much about my family, frustration that is now making me numb. For I have learned those words have helped shield my grandmother from pain and regret, as if their spirits would come back to haunt her and me.

From losing her home to a cyclone to struggling to put food on the table, her life's wounds still are fresh. And this American-born girl, this *ti ameriken,* who in recent years has professed a committed interest in Haiti, has no right—I suppose—to expect my grandmother to accommodate my curiosity as to her life before coming to America, the promised land, where money could supposedly be found on the streets and in public fountains, ready for the taking. When she got off that plane from Port-au-Prince nearly thirty years ago, she left behind a part of herself. And I cannot blame her for discarding a painful past. But it is not only her life she is guarding, it is mine as well, one that is filled with gaps and vague accounts of things, information scooped up along the years through passing mentions and aunts' conversations at the kitchen table. I can't get my grandmother to even mention my late grandfather's name above a whisper. Jotting down his name on pieces of paper helps me to envision this faceless man. I keep his name written in all my journals—otherwise I would forget.

During my college years in Florida, I would beg my grandmother to speak onto the blank cassette tapes that I sent her. But they would go unrecorded, collecting dust on top of the refrigerator. Our phone conversations would be full of awkward pauses when I would ask questions about her life, about how she had raised my own mother in a southern town in Haiti that is surrounded by breadfruit trees, about raising eight children for a man who lived in another house with his wife and children in that very same neighborhood. How my mother barely knew that man. She only would see and smell the cologne-scented man in the white linen suit, who would come by for late evening supper.

"I'll explain everything to you some day," my grandmother insists, changing the subject as she sits in her well-worn leather easy chair, for hours. That day has never come. Her silence infected my mother, my father, my aunts and uncles. They all share something that is unspeakable: our family's history. Sad stories are not good to be passed down from generation to generation, my mother reasons, siding with her mother who didn't tell her much either.

The only time I could get people in my family to speak freely about their past was when a relative would come back from Haiti, bearing gifts. I don't remember when I came to realize how important it was to receive these items: food, liquor, embroidered cotton bed sheets, even a pair of plastic slippers. But I now know those things helped them to remember where they came from, to relive their cherished memories. For it was through those items that I was able to catch glimpses of a sweet and bitter Haiti, of my grandmother and parents. The bites of molasses candy packed with cashews, the sips of egg yolk liquor, the spices, loosened their tongues and they would speak about hunting for pheasants, horseback riding, and summers spent on family farms. My parents would tell us fragmented stories from their childhoods. Pasts that were broken in tiny pieces just like the jars that carried the pickled peppers and fine-shredded cabbage soaked in white distilled vinegar, the fiery odor clinging to the gift-bearers' shirts. Of my father's father abandoning his five children to start another family in neighboring Santo Domingo or Havana, Cuba. No one is really certain where he ended up. Only thing that is for sure is that he came back to Haiti, dying of cancer, so that his children, the ones who made it to America, could bury him. It was as if the odors wafting from the soaked, rickety suitcase brought to our home stirred memories in my parents' minds that were otherwise kept buried deep. In their new lives, in their home on a street called Phillips on the South Side of Chicago, these items served as a truth potion that helped soothe their ripped hearts, as they were transplanted to new jobs where they swept up powdered gum at a Wrigley factory and lifted sharp, cold iron parts at a steel mill.

"You realize how much you miss everything," one family member explained. "How life hasn't been what you expected it to be."

Now that I live on my own, catching my family reflecting on their lives is rare. Instead, when we get together now, we sit at tables, talking about who got married, when will I get married, and who is sick. Superficial topics I can easily discuss with the strangers I now interview. Aside from blood, my family is not connected by much else. Not like a Korean friend of mine, who at a young age was given a book about his lineage that spans thirty-three generations. That's a lot of history, permanence, and family pride. I, on the other hand, cannot even break the silence past my own mother's generation. However, I have jotted down notes, and bits and pieces of stories. And I fill blank cassettes daily on my job, fill them with stories. None of them my own.

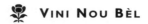

🌸 Vini Nou Bèl

Annie Grégoire

A few months after the assassination of Dr. Martin Luther King, Jr., I was born in a Brooklyn hospital during a hot summer. Early in my life, my father introduced me to the civil-rights leader, for a picture of Dr. King hung on the living room wall of my parents' one-bedroom apartment in Crown Heights, Brooklyn. Although my father never spoke to me about why he displayed a picture of the slain activist next to that of John F. Kennedy in our home, I later came to understand the significance of their portraits.

In elementary school, I started to understand that the portrait of Martin Luther King, Jr. symbolized the struggle for racial equality. During Black History Month, my classmates and I sang "We shall overcome" as loudly as we could and recited poems resonating, "I have a dream . . ." Still, honoring Black History Month had a somber tone, not as exciting to me as the other cultural events celebrated at my bilingual public school. With great anticipation, I looked forward to celebrating Haitian Flag Day at school.

On Haitian Flag Day I always felt special marching in the auditorium wearing my Haitian folkloric attire, a red bandanna covering my head and a blue dress tucked in at the waist with a red scarf, while chanting the national anthem of Haiti. That was the only time

I truly believed I was no different from my peers, as we all marched in unison, showing off the same colors of blue and red. My Haitian-born parents were there singing along with me while we paraded down the aisle. Celebrating Haitian history and culture at this elementary school seemed to foster a great sense of ethnic pride among many students in the French and Spanish bilingual programs, including the few students who were neither of Haitian nor Hispanic descent.

Other times, however, some of my schoolmates, notably the boys, reminded me that I was different. Instead of addressing me as "Annie" they preferred to call me "Blackie." Their teasing began to sound natural, since the term "Blackie" was often used by black people to describe their darker peers. Although I learned to tolerate the taunting, I was somewhat confused about how dark a person needed to be in order to be called "Blackie" since many of the individuals who belittled me were just a shade or two lighter.

As my preteen years approached, I wanted to interact more with young people of different cultural backgrounds. I grew tired of studying French and celebrating Haitian Flag Day. One day I convinced my parents to enroll me in a Catholic grammar school attended by some of the children living on my block. I was hoping to start anew. To my dismay, attention to my dark hue followed me to Catholic school. On the first day of class at my new school, I was greeted with loud laughter by a group of boys sitting in the back of the classroom. Thereafter, one of the boys from that group, who was of Jamaican descent, also chose not to address me as "Annie." This time my new name was "Crispy." He stopped calling me "Crispy" the day I exploded in Language Arts class and cried out loud before all my classmates. From then on, he referred to me by my proper name. The insults by some of the other students did not end though. Occasionally, I was "the Creature from the Black Lagoon" or the child whose mamma left her "in the toaster too long." One time a female classmate snidely remarked, "It's getting darker in here," as I entered the classroom and when I was leaving she said, "It's getting lighter in here." A girl with fair complexion asked me one day, "Do you ever wish you were light-skinned?"

At this grammar school, I did have the opportunity to make more friends of different cultural backgrounds: African-American, Trinidadian, Irish, Italian, Puerto Rican, and others. But there was also a large student population of Haitian descent. Being of Haitian descent at my school brought little pride and prestige, however. The 1980s rolled in with the rise of the AIDS epidemic, linking the disease to Haitians. Meanwhile, numerous Haitians were fleeing their homeland in shabby boats to reach American shores. Unfortunately, the Haitian-American students were not exempt from being stigmatized even in a school in which they dominated. Some students pretended they couldn't speak a word of Haitian *Kreyòl* while others tried to distance themselves from their Haitian-born parents, identifying themselves as Americans.

From grammar school, I moved on to a high school with a mixed student population of African, European, Hispanic, and Asian origins. Although the different ethnic groups were tolerant of one another, they hardly intermingled. Occasionally I heard "ethnic jokes" told by students of various groups, but I was only truly affected by the derogatory remarks about dark-skinned blacks or people of Haitian descent. In high school, I purposely stayed away from the lunchroom and tried to avoid the comments by taking unpopular and extra classes and working in the school office.

It was not until I entered college that I faced prejudice from some white students and experienced racial discrimination and tensions between black and white people. Dealing with the race issue and black-white relations helped me to better understand the seeds of narrow-mindedness while shedding light on the reasons behind the class and color politics among many black people. The summer after my sophomore year, I studied in Rome. I was the only black person in my program. In Italy, I was so self-conscious that my eyes often dropped as I saw individuals pointing me out in a crowd. I also learned about prejudices within the Italian community, mainly the negative views that southern and northern Italians have about each other. Some southern Italians saw their northern fellow citizens as snooty city dwellers; whereas certain northern Italians looked down at their southern counterparts as lowly peasants or *"terroni."*

A year later, I embarked on another adventure: I went to study in Paris. The week before I left for France, Yusuf Hawkins, a black teenager, was killed by a group of white youths in Brooklyn. At the time, hoping to find solace in the "City of Light," Yussef's death left me indifferent. Unfortunately, France, like all nations, has its share of social problems. Because of my color, I had to obtain the tenants' special approval before moving into an apartment. Likewise, most people in France assumed that I was either domestic help residing in the maid's chamber; an African-American student who loved jazz and came from Harlem; or a Senegalese immigrant to France. Even Senegalese greeted me in Wolof and often seemed insulted that I did not speak their language. There was also some tension between the West African and West Indian communities in France. Based on many conversations with members of both communities, a mutual resentment suggested tension between them. While a number of Africans believed that Francophone West Indians tended to promote their European or Indian ancestry while denying their African roots, some West Indians, particularly Guadeloupians and Martinicans, felt that the African presence in France was a reminder of past slavery and present colonization. Strangers often called out *"Africaine!"* when I walked by. To retaliate, I proudly let them know of my Haitian heritage, reminding them of the Caribbean colony France had lost through a slave revolt. Ignorance also dwelt in the minds of some American students in the study-abroad program. I was feasting on a French delicacy in a Parisian café when an American female student of Hispanic descent scornfully referred to Haitian *Kreyòl* as a "tribal language." Sometimes it seemed safer to simply identify myself as "American." Consequently, during my year in France, I was accused by many different groups of people of lying about my nationality and not being proud to be African. By the time I left Paris, I was very confused about who I was.

All the while, strong racial tensions were brewing in New York City. Reactions to the killing of Yusuf Hawkins, the election of New York City's first black mayor, and the Food and Drug Administration's controversial policy banning Haitians from donating blood in the United States were intensifying. In April 1990, thousands of Haitians marched across the Brooklyn Bridge together, protesting the FDA's policy of labeling Haitians as AIDS carriers. Ironically, the AIDS stigma helped to create a sense of unity among Haitians, transcending social and ethnic backgrounds. Although I was in France at the time, my heart was in New York City that day.

With the arrival of the 1990s, a resurgence of Afrocentric fads in fashion, movies, and music began to appear in urban America: the music of Soul II Soul and Public Enemy; Afrocentric accessories prominent in Spike Lee's films. Lee's socially conscious films helped to expose color and class issues in the black community as well as race relations in America, particularly in New York City. During this revival of black pride, I went from being called "Blackie" and "Crispy" to "Chocolate" and "Dark and Lovely." While I didn't especially find being compared to an edible treat or a brand name of a hair relaxer to be a compliment, at that point I was ready to deal with my feelings of inferiority because of being dark-skinned.

Upon returning to college, I immediately joined the Haitian Student Organization, which had received a negative reputation on campus for protesting the Blood Drive. Learning that the FDA's policy had also banned Americans of Haitian descent from donating blood, I began to question the value of my American citizenship. With the approach of the Persian Gulf War, the U.S. federal government finally listened to the anger of the Haitian community and lifted the ban in December 1990.

The years after college graduation marked a major transition in my life. I had been so busy evaluating myself by people's perceptions of my skin color and ethnic background that I didn't seriously think about what I truly wanted to do with my life. After three years of working at the United Nations, I decided to become a teacher. Strangely, I first taught French at a Catholic high school in Brooklyn attended by a large student population of Haitian descent. Like me, most of these students were American-born of Haitian parentage. They were also proud of their Haitian heritage, often chatting in Haitian *Kreyòl*. While blurting out the lyrics of the latest hip-hop songs, many of them teased one another in the language of their Haitian-born parents. However, the black students at this Catholic high school, whether Haitian or non-Haitian, were still influenced by the color-conscious sentiments of their peers and those who had come before them. I occasionally heard and saw some students being teased about the darkness of their skin; a few still compared the tint of the inner surface of their forearms to determine their true hue. I then realized that cultural pride went beyond one's language, history, traditions, customs, and ethnic makeup. I thought about the irony of Haitian history: the first independent black nation to successfully revolt against oppression and yet, among some of us feelings of inferiority still lurk, keeping Haitians of different classes and skin tones divided.

Although my father was greatly inspired by Dr. Martin Luther King's fight for racial equality, he had already internalized the belief that black people had limitations and could only succeed in certain fields. My father was very disappointed that I had become a teacher, believing that teaching was not prestigious and brought little wealth. Even after I earned a master's degree in foreign language education, my father still wasn't impressed, hoping that I would one day fulfill his dream of becoming a doctor. A few months after receiving my graduate degree, I lost my grandmother and my father; they passed away a few weeks apart. In 1998, a few months after their deaths, I went on a journey to Haiti for the first time. During the time I was there, I reflected on my late grandmother's words, *"Vini nou bèl, ale nou lèd."* My grandmother believed that our arrival on Earth was beautiful, but our departure from Earth was the contrary. Yet, her passing inspired me to finally visit Haiti; for she had a great love for her country.

I saw so much poverty and injustice in Haiti, but I also watched Haitians who were struggling and surviving despite these limitations. In Haiti, I visited my grandmother's and great-grandmother's homes. Painted in bright pastel colors, their houses stood in the middle of a grassy field surrounded by fruitful plants. There I was also introduced to my mother's cattle, branded with her initials. In the swarming heat, I sat with my cousins, who reminisced about their memorable childhoods in Haiti on our family's land as well as their escapades riding into town on mules and donkeys. I imagined myself climbing the Haitian mountains while carrying heavy baskets atop my head; I envisioned myself bathing in flowing streams while others washed their clothes in the rivers. Nevertheless, my imagination inevitably turned to reality as I remember the people struggling in their daily lives. Wading in the warm, clear-blue waters along a Haitian beach resort, I found comfort in knowing that my mother and siblings were still present in my life.

Overcoming my insecurity about my dark skin has been my greatest obstacle. I have always been proud of my Haitian background, never ashamed of my Haitian roots; never hiding my Haitian identity whenever the topic of AIDS emerged; never silencing the African sounds of the Haitian *Kreyòl*; never feeling disgraced by the Haitian refugees who were risking their lives in choppy waters to come to the United States. Likewise, I have always found warmth in embracing the spiritual drive of black people. However, for a long time, believing that my dark skin was inferior often prevented me from living openly; walking along the beach; dancing wantonly at school parties; feeling attractive in a deep red dress; or laughing at someone's joke. Keeping quietly to myself, I hoped to attract as little attention as possible.

Becoming a teacher has been therapeutic for me, helping me to feel more comfortable in my skin. This has helped me to foster confidence and self-esteem in elementary-age students, particularly black students. As a result of working with young people who have greater obstacles to face than the shade of their skin, I am more concerned with preparing children to gain a keener understanding of social problems inherent in all societies—intolerance, war, illiteracy, hunger, poverty, health issues, environmental troubles, abuse, and violence. Every day as I stand before these students, my greatest hope is that they will learn to see beyond stereotypes and misconceptions, respecting each other for who they are as human beings.

🌹 HOME IS . . .

Sophia Cantave

I've thought about going home, collapsing into my mother's arms and asking her, without speaking, to comfort me, to tell me that the bad world won't get me. But I know that if I go home—yeah, she'll hold me for a few seconds, but then she'll let out a sigh, with that look in her eyes, that look of decades of working, and worrying and she'll say, "Daughter, since you've been gone . . ." beginning her own narrative before I can say, "Manman, I'm tired of being alone. I don't speak their language. They don't understand me." But then I would remember that our vocabulary never included words to explain my loneliness or my sense of fear and if I suddenly started crying because of an unspeakable loss, she would offer to do whatever she could to make me "happy" again. In the end I would say "I'm fine really. That was nothing. I'm just tired." In this way, our vocabulary never expanded. I would take a deep breath and suck in the tears, the fear, the reason why I came home in the first place, and listen to her instead. Afterward, I would prepare to go back to the world, still feeling lost and alone despite her promise to pray for me and a reminder to keep the Notre Dame amulet on me always. I would go back into the world with the overwhelming desire to turn around and say "Manman, I still don't speak their language." But home and my mother's arms were always beyond reach and unable to hold me for very long because we had never really developed a vocabulary to discuss what was asked of me.

I wrote these words on the back page of Barbara Johnson's *Wake of Deconstruction* on October 16, 1994, during my first semester in graduate school. Suddenly, in a theory class about language, I found myself without a true language of my own. In previous environments, ones that called for a different English, I had responded by code switching, quickly learning the jargon and hastily falling in line. This was an invaluable skill and one that I knew, even as early as seventh grade, could push me beyond the limitations of Fifth Avenue, Brooklyn—where I grew up the daughter of Haitian immigrants—to the halls of higher learning at Tufts University. Of course, there was a sacrifice. Only years later would I seriously think about what my sacrifice had been: my mother tongue. I wasn't sure if that language was *Kreyòl*. I just knew I needed to speak something that had eluded me for years. English was not my mother tongue, but I made myself believe it was. I could not remember a time when I didn't speak English.

Il n'y a pas de text. There is no text. This small French sentence had become all the rage. I had lived with this concept my whole adult life and suddenly I didn't want to anymore. *Il n'y a pas de text* seemed to clash with my translation of the French words on the Haitian flag: *L'union fait la force*. In union, there is strength. I set about writing myself into being.

Going through the journals and letters I've written over the years, I see myself expressing over and over the same anxiety about language, the quest to maintain some essential part of myself while shape-shifting and searching for total fluidity. Making simultaneous translations for myself of everything from ways to speak to my mother to the creed on Haiti's flag, I felt myself floating between fragments that I was always rearranging. To keep track of these fragments, I kept journals. I believed then and now that the written word, in whatever form, would ground me and make my fragmented self whole. The words I wrote in my journal were inscribed in secret. These were words I rarely shared with my family, words that I hid even harder once my father asked to know what it was that I was always writing about. I would have had to read it to him and then do the translation. The English that he and my mother had encouraged me to speak and perfect also helped to increase the distance between us.

The truth hit me in theory class one day: I was not just a black girl but a Haitian girl and for the first time I longed for home and home was a bunch of people and a culture I knew by name, accepted at face value, but did not know intimately. Using the back pages of Johnson's *Wake,* I sent a psychic call to my mother, imagining that only she could explain why I didn't speak anybody's language. I sent out the call and heard my own voice ask why I didn't have any way to *speak* to my mother about my loss and all that was tearing at me.

I was not blaming my mother but searching for a mother tongue. I had surprised even myself with the words I'd scribbled out of frustration and fear in the back of Johnson's book. I was admitting that my mother and I did not speak the same language and yet I knew that it was my language barrier, not hers, that kept us from understanding each other. I wanted to find a bridge; I wanted to learn to speak a forgotten tongue.

August 1997 Journal Entry:
I have always had language issues, have always felt that my voice leaves too much room for misunderstandings, misinterpretations. Having to always negotiate when and where to use my voice often left important things about me unsaid. I think of Billie Holliday with all her problems, living in fragments, breaking down and whispering "Hush now, don't explain." Not having to explain myself or create whole new fictions about who I am or what I want is what I long for, like Billie.

But in my journals I keep trying to explain me, my Haitian family, and our place in this country. Before I started graduate school, my mother asked me when I was going to visit "my country." It took me a moment to realize that she meant Haiti, the place we had all migrated from when I was five years old. Until then, I had never realized that Haiti was a place that people returned to. It was never spoken of except as a place people left or from which they had to be sent for. Rarely did my mother talk about the daughters that she had left behind in Haiti, sisters I remembered vaguely or not at all. All my life, Haiti had seemed an even more distant, mythical place than the lost Africa of African Americans. I never denied being Haitian-born, but it also made sense for me to be considered an African American. After all, Haiti is in the Americas and I am of African descent. Only I knew more about African America than I did about Haiti. In graduate school, I was pursuing formal training in African-American literature, history, and culture. I had mistakenly believed that being Haitian didn't require formal study or inquiry. Haiti was in my name and in my home. Only I kept going farther and farther away from home and I hadn't yet learned how to go back and choose what to hold on to and what to let go of. A crisis was inevitable—and since I had been studying words and language, my crisis came in the classroom. After all those years, I still did not own a particular language. I had to go back to my beginning, yet I didn't want the academic in me to turn my personal dilemma into research. This journey was going to come by way of my mother. I had to humbly step down from my scholarly perch to see what my people could give me—if I asked. To begin fixing my language problem, I had to do the impossible, return home and "step in the same river twice."

I had left home to get a degree and now I wanted to return. I knew it would sound crazy to people who spoke heavily accented

English, who often had to ask their children to translate for them or accompany them on appointments that required "good" English. In my family, going back never seemed to be an option. Going back home without a degree was unimaginable. For all my parents' hard work, they needed the children of the new country to do things they'd only dreamed of. I was the first of the new, the fifth child of both my parents but their first together. I had to do more than Fifth Avenue, Sunset Park, Brooklyn allowed and surpass their tentative dreams.

Once I caught myself wondering if my mother ever had dreams that didn't include being the caretaker of a large splintered family. I wondered if she constantly talked to herself like I talked to myself about my future, about the path that I wanted to choose for myself instead of what was expected of me. I was afraid of what I would find out; it was easier to plan in secret for my future than to ask her about her hopes as a girl.

I knew my father conflated U.S. schools with what he remembered of Haitian schools. In his Haiti, school was reserved for the selected few. I knew that my father never forgave his father for forcing him to stop his formal education in order to work. At the beginning of my senior year in high school, out of love and duty, my father had sat me down and said, "Sophia, you can go to whatever college you want."

My heart had contracted and I said "I can?" He took my hand in his and said, "Yes, any college in Brooklyn, Manhattan, Queens, anywhere the bus or the train can take you." My heart had plunged. The world I wanted was bigger than the five boroughs my father offered me.

I'd worked on my applications to faraway colleges at school and forged his and my mother's signatures where necessary. In the spring I received a letter of acceptance from my first choice university in

Boston and took that as a sign that I was meant to leave. I'd shared the good news with my teachers and friends. So I wouldn't back out, I'd told my mother. I needed her on my side so she could rally the various family members to speak on my behalf. I still had to be the one to tell my father of my decision to leave his house and go beyond the perimeters he had set for me.

Once I'd told him, two months passed before my father spoke to me again, but when he did he gave his consent. We sat down in his room and he told me that he knew I was a good girl, that I was going to school to study and better myself. I agreed. I had won. Afterward I did something that few Haitian girls my age did: I attended my senior prom and at my father's suggestion arranged to sleep over at my best friend's house to avoid traveling alone late that night. Only when I got to sleep away from home—a serious no-no—did I understand my victory. My father and mother were letting me go.

If I didn't know how to speak to my family before, I certainly couldn't speak to them now. I'd never learned how to talk to my family without being on guard, without always preparing to counteract my father's No in some way. No, *Il n'y a pas de text* could not explain my foreignness that first year away from home, nor could it explain the place my parents called Fifth Avenue, Brooklyn but I knew as Sunset Park. Back then I wanted to escape the fate of never knowing what I was capable of because I was black, because I was a Haitian girl, because I was poor. That overwhelming desire sustained me through the college years. But in graduate school, I suddenly needed to talk to my mother about what it meant to actually escape. I wanted to speak to her of what I had spent my whole life unconsciously running from: her powerlessness.

During one of my tirades against my family, my mother once asked me, "If we are these terrible things, then what are you?" Only

now can I say, I am my mother. I am my father. I am Fifth Avenue—
also known as Sunset Park—Brooklyn. And to do what life and
graduate school requires of me, I need to make peace with that. I
need to learn to speak with a different part of myself. I no longer
write unmailed letters to my mother. I call her and tell her things I
didn't know I could say.

During the 1995–96 school year, I went looking for Haitians outside of my family. My whole life I'd never had one Haitian friend.
I decided to volunteer my Saturday mornings with other Haitian
women mentoring Haitian girls who reminded me of myself. Looking back I wondered what, if anything, the great thinkers like Der-
rida, De Man, Foucault, or Johnson could say that didn't seem to
mock me and the things I had done, the circular search I had been
on, had always been on, in language. How could they account for
what I knew about living in shadows, in crevices, dying each time
I remade myself, surviving in gaps or waiting on that one elliptical
mark for a space to enter.

There are people whose spirits are destroyed by not being able to
conquer a language, people like my parents for example. They speak
in heavily accented English, and must sometimes use their children's
voices instead of their own. They do not get to talk about their
experiences but hope that their children will even things out in the
future and make them right. Perhaps my mother had given birth to
me so that I could do all the things that she never did. Only now,
as I learn to speak forgotten words, am I beginning to understand
her bravery. Even among new Haitian friends, some encountered in
Boston and others while I spent hours on the prettiest Haitian beach,
in the prettiest Haitian sea, I find myself mourning, for her and for
myself. Perhaps to really make things right, I have to accept my own
version of Haiti, to become my own Haitian daughter.

🌸 MAP VIV: MY LIFE AS A NYABINGHI RAZETTE

Marie Nadine Pierre

I am a Nyabinghi Razette. Most people identify me as a Rastafarian. The Nyabinghi was an army of women and men brought together by Haile Selassie I, the Emperor of Ethiopia, to fight oppression. Among Rastafarians, Nyabinghi means "death to all oppressors." Razette was coined by Sistren Jahzinine and it refers to a female Rastafarian. As a Nyabinghi Rastafarian, I believe in the divinity of Haile Selassie I and the Empress Menen.

My life as a Nyabinghi Razette has not earned me friends nor has it brought me wealth. However it has connected me even more to my Haitian self and has given me the aesthetic and spiritual freedom that I have always sought. Some people feel that a Haitian cannot be a Rastafarian. I don't see any contradiction between my lifestyle as a Rastafarian and my ethnic identity as a Haitian. Those who do not see the obvious parallels between us have a narrow view of both Haitians and Rastafarians.

Perhaps the closest analogy that can be drawn between Haitians and Rastafarians is through spirituality. Haitians and Rastafarians share spiritual paths (*Vodou* and RastafarI) that have roots in Africa and that continue to act as positive forces in the world. Members of the African diasporas from different countries practice their own

171

forms of spirituality such as Obeah, Condomble, and Santería, just as there are different groups of Rastafarians, from the Twelve Tribe Rastas to the Nazarite Rastas.

Another issue that promotes the separatist view between Haitians and Rastafarians is language. In the Rastafarian *trod*, or lifestyle, the English language is prominent. Irits, the Rastafarian language, which is not to be confused with Jamaican patois, is overly influenced by English to the extent of drowning out other languages such as Haitian *Kreyòl*. I am often appalled at the ethnocentric perspective of some English-speaking Rastafarians who go to great lengths to discredit and discourage other languages, especially Haitian *Kreyòl*. A transnational Haitian, I was born in the United States and spent my formative years (age one through eleven) in Haiti; I speak English well enough so that it is relatively easier for me to adapt to Irits. At the same time, I have to recognize that Irits is one way that most non-*Kreyòl*-speaking Rastas identify themselves as other-than-Haitian.

In spite of these struggles in and outside of the *trod*, my faith as a Nyabinghi Rastafarian could never cancel out my identity as a Haitian. I love Haitian music: *mizik rasin, konpa*; Haitian food: *diri kole* and *bannan peze*. Now, as a vegan who does not eat meat, I cook brown rice with peas and I eat tofu and seitan instead of *griyo* and *boulèt*. In fact, my version of Ital, or Rastafarian cooking, is Haitian food with vegan substitutes. By adopting an Ital or vegan lifestyle, I am fighting the diseases that have plagued many people in my life, including family members, friends, and acquaintances, who have suffered from diabetes, high blood pressure, and heart failure. Without forcing my lifestyle on anyone, I do think that a Rastafarian vegan diet might help many Haitians in the United States who are living under stressful conditions in crowded urban centers in New York, Boston, and Miami or are adjusting from a familiar tropical climate to a cold foreign one.

One of the most treasured manifestations of my life as a Razette and as a Haitian is expressing my love of colors, especially in fabrics, in dresses and skirts, as in the regal dress and headwear that African women wear. I love to wrap my dreadlocks in a beautiful festive Afrocentric fabric, praying for strength as I do from my African and Haitian ancestors.

During Nyabinghis, when Rastafarians gather to chant praises or Isis to the Empress and Emperor of Ethiopia, men are asked to uncover their dreadlocks while women are asked to cover theirs. When I was a "bald head" or had not yet become a Nyabinghi Razette, I thought that black people, including Haitians, who read the Bible were being brainwashed into accepting white domination. However, as a Razette, I became aware of the fact that many of the people described in the Bible, including the Queen of Sheba, King Solomon, and Jesus, are black Africans. Since contemporary scientific evidence shows that civilization began on the African continent, it follows then that Eve's and Adam's descendants would be black.

RastafarI, provides me with a space to explore such ideas. Being a Razette gives me the spiritual freedom to create and re-create myself as a woman of physical and spiritual strength and power. My identity as a transnational Nyabinghi Razette, Haitian, working-class, dark-skinned black woman, doctoral candidate, mother, and wife is best captured by the creative and artistic framework of the collage that joins me not only to the immediate Haitian *dyaspora* in the United States, but to the larger African community all over the world.

My life as a Nyabinghi Razette encourages me to seek the truth about the condition of all black Africans on earth. Both as a Razette and a Haitian, my goal has always been to be free and to be myself. Both as a Razette and a Haitian, I want to live with the truth that black people have been the makers and builders of strong and beautiful civilizations. And they will continue to be.

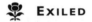 **EXILED**

Sandy Alexandre

I was twelve years old when I was tricked into exile. One weekday morning, as I was preparing to catch the school bus, my mother confronted me with her latest finding in what was then my burgeoning delinquency problem. Because I had neglected to cover the pot of rice from last night's dinner, the cockroaches had easily invaded and spoiled our leftovers. We quarreled: She blamed; I denied. And suddenly, forgetting to whom I was speaking, I made the horrible mistake of responding to one of her comments with the expletive "So?" In retrospect, I must have said the word with too strong a hint of exasperation, with too much of the sense that I had grown quickly inconvenienced by her diatribe. Not only had I said "So?" I had dramatized it by rolling my big insolent eyes. She had never liked that word *so*; she thought it was too curt, too arrogant, and too defiant. The word had no Haitian equivalent to which she could relate, against which she could measure its power. Especially now that it was being used in the context of an argument, she felt safe in assuming the worst of a word whose meaning she did not completely understand. *"Pa di'm so,"* she said as she turned to stare at me in utter disbelief and disgust. "Don't tell me *so*," she repeated. "Do I look like one of your cronies that you can speak to me in such a

174

disrespectful way?" My mother and I had been having many arguments like this one lately, but this dispute finally brought our conflict
to a crisis.

She had had enough of my attitude. She deemed me too Amer-
icanized—too saucy—to handle. Her Haitian upbringing (the ruler
by which she measured good and evil) could no longer tolerate such
unfilial behavior, so she threatened to punish me by sending me back
to New York to live with my father. She warned that as soon as I
returned home from school, I would find my bags packed and ready
for me to be sent away. The sauciness lingered: "Good!" I retorted.
"I don't like Florida anyway!" Not taking her threat seriously, I
sauntered off to school with an air of cool defiance. But because of
the argument, I knew I had missed my bus and so looked more the
fool than the victor I wanted to be; to save some face, I walked out
of the house singing, "I love New York, I love New York" to the
tune of a commercial jingle that she and I both knew. Clearly, my
eyes were not the only things on a roll!

When I returned home, sure enough, my mother handed me my
luggage and then, along with my uncle, drove me to the airport.
Walking through the airport, I summoned the same cool saunter of
nonchalance that allowed me to keep my dignity only a few hours
before. But underneath that so cool exterior lay a completely incred-
ulous and regretful prodigal daughter. How could I be so foolish?
How can she be so serious? She's blown this thing out of proportion.
Does she really mean to send me away? Am I really all that bad? Why
must I always be so rebellious? Why does the sign over my flight gate
read: DEPARTURE TO PORT-AU-PRINCE, HAITI?

In the fifteen minutes before I was to board the plane, my mother,
with a smug smile of victory, explained that I was actually going to
be living with her sister in Haiti. Her announcement was the "Ta
da!" of a magician whose craft was more entertaining to himself than

to his audience. So, while she was being thrilled by her own perspicacity, I couldn't see the humor nor appreciate the genius behind the trick of changing flight destinations. Although her decision was obviously final, I was too shocked to accept the reality that she had proudly unveiled before me. I was in a state of denial. I found her reasons neither sufficient nor strong enough to justify my punishment: "It's for your own good; You're too much, too incorrigible." And the inevitable, "Children in Haiti don't disrespect their elders. You'll learn from them," she predicted, "to comport yourself as a child." Those oft-referred-to "children in Haiti" had some nerve, to keep reminding my mother of how horrible a child I was. How tired I was of hearing my mother sing the praises of these Haitian angels! But soon, whether I liked it or not, I was also going to be—if even just superficially—a child of Haiti.

When it dawned on me that I had been so cleverly deceived, that I was indeed going to Haiti, a place I imagined had no bathrooms, no refrigerators, and no English, I started to cry and then to scream out of sheer terror. Through my tear-glazed eyes, I spied a flight attendant who had a look of grave concern and pity; so, choosing fight over flight (pun intended), I grabbed the opportunity to try to save myself from banishment.

"Don't cry," she said. "What's wrong?"

Pointing to my uncle as if he were the guilty one in a criminal line-up, I sobbed: "He's not my father! He's (gasp for air and then a phlegmful sniff-sniff) not my father!" I wanted to convey the impression that I was being abducted by a complete stranger. My pointing, trembling, finger and my crying eyes combined to form a plea for help, to make me a paragon of victimization. Save me! I exuded.

You can imagine the commotion that my outburst caused. The flight attendant was as horrified as I had predicted. I knew that I could appeal to the sensibilities of an America that, at the time, wanted the children on its milk cartons found and their kidnappers prosecuted. Certainly, she was not going to stand idly by while, right before her very eyes, I became an "unsolved mystery."

To this day, I am still surprised at the desperate measures to which I lowered myself to save myself from Haiti. But this tactic only helped to stall the expulsion process. The exile must go on! My mother quickly explained the situation and after everyone was mollified, the attendant escorted me to my seat. I had been defeated.

Had I known then what I know now, I would have understood both the comedy and the import behind the situation in which I found myself, for on the plane I was surrounded by symbols that marked my situation as a potentially profound, enlightening, and extraordinary one. To my right, on the seat beside me, sat a middle-aged Haitian woman who was deeply embittered about the ruckus that I had caused. She was "familiar with my kind," and with a sort of "fire and brimstone" speech that she seemed to have saved for this moment, she accused me of being an ingrate, a child too ripe for my age, a Haitian American gone too American. Indeed, she knew me too well! As if she had been planted on the plane by my mother, she continued to torment me about the many ways in which my punishment was justified. That my plane instead of heading north was flying south seemed ironically appropriate—Haiti was to be my Hades. I knew her "kind" too, and her finding pleasure in my plight made me decide that I didn't like her too much.

To my left sat a Haitian man in his early thirties, who confessed—with a hint of pride—that he himself had been in my present predicament when he was just a young boy going through his adolescent, *vagabon* stage. "When I got to Haiti, I sold all of my clothes and returned to the States. Don't worry, you can do the same thing," he advised. So while Mrs. Fire and Brimstone castigated, I wondered if my mother had packed my favorite green-and-black dress. I could get a lot of money for that one, I assured myself. How symbolic was my seating arrangement—between the good on the right and the not so good on the left. This exile was a parable in the making!

When I arrived in Port-Au-Prince, I was immediately met by my uncle Yvero. "Sandee!" he called out as he rushed over to help me with my bags. "Your mother told me all about your coming." He smiled as he said this, and even though I felt miserable, I couldn't help but smile back at his genuine happiness to see me. Did he know why I had been sent? Would I be able to continue relying on his reassuring smile or would he turn against me—the ingrate, juvenile delinquent—when he discovered my reason for being here? His smile comforted me but it also renewed my sense of shame. I knew that I didn't deserve to be smiled at. I sought no comfort because I was too tired and defeated. I sought no comfort because I refused to believe that there was any to be found in Haiti. If I were never going to see America again, at least I could wallow in the familiar territory of self-pity. But, this was only temporary, because I had resigned myself to exile; that is, I had surrendered. I had no other choice. It was clear to me that if I wanted to survive in Haiti, I could choose to be neither arrogant nor disobedient. That I needed to acculturate myself for survival purposes necessitated that I substitute humility for impudence, respect for disrespect and acceptance for denial. I was now in a situation and a place where I could not allow my Americanness to override whatever Haitianness I possessed. I needed to tap into all the Haitian resources that I owned because I was going to be here for an undefined amount of time. My title of "American" meant nothing good in this country. My uncle knew why I was here: I was here because there was a correlation between there being something wrong with America and there being something wrong with me.

Uncle Yvero rushed me out of the airport and quickly hailed a tap-tap. He had a commanding and respectable presence. He was younger than my mother and looked it, with his thick head of black hair and well-kempt mustache that complemented it. He carried himself, and my bags, with masculine ease. I felt safe in his company. If I wasn't careful, his strength would ruin me. After all, I wasn't here to depend on someone else's Haitianness; I was here to find my own.

He offered me a Chiclet. "*Ki jan ou ye?*" he asked.

"*M pa pi mal*"—I'm fine—I answered. After an hour or so, we transferred to another tap-tap headed to our destination—Arcahaie. When we finally arrived, it was already night. I knew we were in the country somewhere because it was pitch black everywhere I looked.

"Sandee?"

"*Wi*," I replied. "I'm right over here."

It was my aunt, Mante Venide. I couldn't actually see her, but I immediately recognized her voice from the cassette recordings that she occasionally sent to my mother. Her greeting was always the same—your name in the form of a question. She had supper waiting for me, she explained. "I know you must be hungry. Here. Eat, child." I did. I ate and then soon after that went to sleep.

Early the very next morning, by the crow of the rooster in residence, my aunt woke me up to introduce me to the family: my cousins Alex and Tififi, my uncle Yvero, my aunt Madam Ka (Kalix) and my uncle Ka and a whole slew of other relatives. "We are your family," she concluded her introduction. "This is your home." And with that, she took my hand and told me that we were going to the market to get some things that she needed. And so began my exile.

My aunt, her brother, and her two children shared two huts in a big yard that also housed some of my other relatives. I was assigned a bed in the room where my cousins slept. Since I was so familiar with tiled floors, angular walls and ceilings, and indoor plumbing, the room seemed unfinished, makeshift. It was cozy and afforded much comfort in its rustic way. Simplicity and frugality defined life in the Haitian countryside. The cobbled floors of the room were layered with very fine dust. Every day my cousins and I took turns sweeping the floor, although I never understood the utility behind such an everlasting chore. No matter how much my cousins, my aunt, or I swept, the floor always remained slightly dusty.

During my stay, my aunt Venide made me help her cook, buy groceries, wash and iron clothes, feed the chickens and the pig, clean the yard, run errands for and keep company with my elderly aunt. Whatever she did, I emulated to the best of my abilities. Whatever I was told to do, I did. I never disliked doing these chores. I approached them as if they were small adventures. I wanted to prove that I was not as American as I had been accused and convicted of being. I felt a sense of kinship when I sat on a small wooden chair beside my aunt and, imitating her, wrapped my thighs around the little ceramic basin in which she washed clothes. She scrubbed the clothes with masterful skill while I, her apprentice, scrubbed like a madwoman for want of that skill. Under her expert hands, the clothes squeaked relentlessly as if to complain about the pain they suffered from being scrubbed too vigorously. Mante Venide's pursed lips and deeply furrowed brow told me that she was oblivious to their cries. I liked that our laundry detergent was simply a big block of soap. Everything I used, from the outhouse that threatened to swallow me whole to the bed I slept on, was as unpretentious as my cousins, my family, and our living arrangements. After we were done with the wash, I felt a sense of genuine achievement when I saw our whites gleaming on the rocks we had laid them on to dry. I felt important when I carried water from the well without spilling it.

Like all prisoners, at some point I was even allowed recreation. I got to play games and run reasonably wild with my cousins. We played with marbles; we sang songs; we gossiped about a neighborhood hussy whom I never met; we competed to see who could tell the funniest joke to the pig; we played hide-and-seek, and when we were really bored we teased the dangerous *"Ti Malis"* out of its underground home with cupfuls of water. *"L ap mòde 'ou*—it's going to bite you!" Alex would scream every time the insect showed its annoyed head.

But as acclimated as I may have seemed on the surface, I was still unabashedly American in essentials.

On Sunday morning we went to church. Since I was already familiar with this ritual from my mass-attending Sundays in America, I ironed my favorite green-and-black dress to wear for the occasion. When I went to search my suitcases for a pair of nylon stockings so that I could put the finishing touches to my ensemble, I was annoyed to discover that my mother had not packed a pair for me. I informed my aunt that I could not attend mass without pantyhose. She laughed. It was too hot to wear stockings. I felt wronged and misunderstood. What did practicality or comfort have to do with style? I found her a bit too Haitian, too country, too old-fashioned. My sense of style was being undermined by someone who actually let the weather get in the way of appearance. I was also angry that it was actually hot outside. I knew better than to confront my aunt with my opinions. Because I was still a child, freedom of speech, especially that of dissent, wasn't my right. Unnerved, but still adorned in green-and-black polyester finery, I walked to church alongside my aunt and my cousins. By the time we reached the church, I realized that my dress—unlike anyone else's—bore a sheen that was too immodest, too gaudy for church. I was being loud without having said a word. I stood out when I should have blended in. Bowing my head in prayer, I was glad to discover that my patent leather shoes had turned from conspicuously shiny to humbly dusty. Haiti's dirt redeemed me, but only to embarrass me later that afternoon.

After we had returned home from church and had eaten lunch, my cousins and I went to play hide and seek in the yard. Tififi and I went to hide while Alex counted *un deux trois.* . . . Still unfamiliar with the area, I found it hard to find a place to hide. Alex was already at *quinze* and I was still looking for a hiding place. I began to panic. Spotting a *kenèp* tree, I dashed for cover behind it. As I ran toward the tree, I slipped and fell in a small pool of mud. The first word out of my mouth was "Shit!" Alex and Tififi came running. They laughed and pointed in my direction while Alex kept giggling and repeating the word *shit* over and over again.

I was angry and refused to get up. I was embarrassed for myself and for Alex who, I assumed, would be punished for his imitation of the corrupt, and now contagious, American exile. I lay brooding in the mud. I didn't try to get up. I wanted my aunt to locate the cause of my profane reaction outside of myself. Was it my fault that this part of the yard was so muddy? Maybe if I were more familiar with the yard, I would not have reacted as I did. I relied on my foreignness as an excuse.

Even during the night, surrounded and disguised by utter darkness as I was, I was every bit a foreigner. To my unsympathetic cousins, I had no qualms about revealing my fears of the zombie population that I was certain inhabited Haiti's nights. When my cousins ventured into the yard away from the house to play and tell stories, I pleaded for them to stay on the porch with me. Haiti's nights had a quality that loomed too huge and formidable in relation to my physical size, my naiveté and my city-girl upbringing. The porch was solid and dependable. The nights, on the other hand, were a bit too dark, a bit too quiet . . . a bit too vast and intangible. Haiti's nights made you think that you could have nightmares with your eyes wide open, so that you'd want to close your eyes just to situate yourself in your own darkness—too afraid to blend in and get lost in a darkness that wasn't your own . . . a nightmare that wasn't your own. Here in Haiti, I easily (if even unfairly) equated good and evil with things diurnal and nocturnal. Whenever the sun set, I felt taunted by a darkness that knew me as a foreigner . . . a Haitian darkness that sensed my fears and had no pity for the American me.

For two weeks, my life as a stranger in a strange land continued in this manner. I didn't feel at home. I wanted to go back to school. I wanted to return to my mother.

The Monday following the second week of my stay in Haiti, my uncle Yvero claimed to have received a letter from my mother. "If you think that you have truly reformed, your mother says that she would like you to return home. So do you think that you've reformed?" my uncle asked.

Of course I have, I thought to myself, especially if it means that I can go back home. But for the sake of seeming sincere and apologetic, I hesitated in my response. I wanted my uncle to understand that I was using this moment of silence to reflect on my wrongdoings. Finally after a few minutes I bowed my head in contrition and said, "Wi, I have reformed." And after a long speech from my uncle and my aunt about how lucky I was to have a mother who cared about me and how deeply foolish I was not to cherish and appreciate that fact, I was told to go and say good-bye to the rest of my extended family. I was going to be leaving for Florida the next day. My stint as an exile was over.

Although I am the only girl that I know of who has had such an experience to recount, I am certainly not the only Haitian American who has an exiled-to-Haiti-for-reform story, for I know several

Haitian–American boys who (like me) have been sent to Haiti to change their potentially self-destructive behaviors. Like my mother, the mothers of these young men relied on the tried-and-true effect of stubborn love, pride, and hope to discipline their children. Because we seemed caught in a frenzy to fit in, our mothers attempted to rescue us, if not by superseding, then by tempering the present with the past, the modern with tradition, America with Haiti. With each child that a Haitian mother has to raise in America, she has to deal with the *triple*-consciousness of its Haitian, American, and Black identities. In junior high school, I was known to my black peers as the just-got-off-the-banana-boat refugee or the *Vodou* queen. I fit into neither of their notions of what it means to be Black or American. Out of ignorance of my own culture, I let those insults sting. Out of ignorance of what it truly means to be Haitian, I let those insults define me. Not now. Not ever. Years later, while on a study-abroad trip to China, although I knew no Swahili nor had ever been to Africa, I was referred to as "the African." While visiting one of the autonomous regions in Northern China, I met a little girl who, pointing in my direction, greeted me as "Kunta Kinte"—the protagonist of Alex Haley's *Roots*. The television movie series had just been shown there. My black face summoned the association with the only other black face this little girl had ever seen. I wasn't an individual, nor did the fact that I am female, and Kinte male, matter. I was just Black. In China when I insisted I was American the Chinese raised skeptical eyebrows.

I questioned my identity then, but wouldn't now because of what I've learned about myself. When you come to know and embrace yourself—whether you have two, three, or four identities to reconcile—you understand that you have everything to gain from those experiences that challenge your justifications for being who you say and think you are. In fact, the lessons learned from these experiences help you achieve the power to shape rather than be shaped by your own future experiences.

As extravagant a form of punishment as my exile seems, I've decided that it was most necessary and most justifiable and certainly most Haitian. By being consistently rude to my mother, I demonstrated my ignorance of the value of respecting my parents and, in extension, my elders. I dared to challenge a philosophy of living that is steeped in common sense and tradition. I dared to think that I was immune from Haitian lore and Haitian justice by virtue of being born in the U.S.A. At twelve years old, I became a walking manifestation of an imperialism that my mother would not endure; with every backtalk, head-wag, eye-roll and "So?", I denied, attacked, and decried everything my mother understood to be Haitian. I was a Haitian American trying to suffocate (whether consciously or not) the Haitian part of my identity. My mother would not tolerate this murder of both her culture and my identity.

My mother was always one step ahead of me and my siblings because she parented vigilantly and ceaselessly (and still continues to do so). I am grateful that she was slicker when I was just slick. For each failed attempt at deceiving her or preempting her authority, I grew to realize and finally accept the intrinsic contrast between my role as the bumbling child and her role as the experienced parent. I am grateful that she knew the limits of her own tolerance. How else can a mother diagnose and then treat an intolerable child if she has not first defined, for herself and eventually her children, what is tolerable? I am grateful that she intervened on my behalf every time I showed signs of becoming less than the decent human being that she wanted me and my siblings to be. My mother has given me a story that I love to tell; it is a "Go to your room" story, Haitian-style.

Haitians have a term *"san manman"* that literally means motherless.

But *"san manman"* does not necessarily mean that one doesn't have a mother, but that one behaves as though one didn't have a mother, as if one were raised without guidance, morals, without the principles that perpetuate culture and a strong community.

And it was because of my mother's fear that I was losing or taking for granted these same ancient properties that she sent me to Haiti so that I could reacquaint myself with them. She wanted me to witness, firsthand, those ancient properties of unconditional self-respect and respect for others shown by the paradigmatic "children of Haiti," through the struggles that my aunt endured raising two children in the poor countryside, through the dignity and respect with which they lived their lives despite the odds, through the interactions between mother and child, the elders and the young, the womenfolk and the menfolk.

I've said that my mother has given me a wonderful story, but I must also acknowledge what I understand to have come before that story, what always was, before the story ever began—the moral. My mother started with a moral and had me trace a path to it with my own story. She has given me a lesson of life that I practice every day. I respect my elders and all others not out of terror of further banishment, but out of an understanding of myself in relation to America, Haiti, and the larger world. It would be foolish to think that I had actually reformed after that one exile to Haiti. Of course, I hadn't. It takes more than a "go to your room," even if that room is actually another country, to discipline a child. My understanding came like most do—through a gradual process of trial and error. But I know that I am most fortunate that my mother refused to remain complaisant about her child's moral development.

In a world where insults still exist and still can sting, there must be culture. In a world where only one may parent where two, three, four, and seven used to, there must be history. In a world where fitting in may mean selling out, there must be keepers of the past, reminders of the ancient ways. James Baldwin, who understood the value of the past in sustaining a stable and dignified present, alluded in his *Notes of a Native Son* to his envy of some Haitians' ability to trace their history back to regal roots. There are rewards of dignity, pride, and honor that proceed from being placeable and traceable.

My siblings and I didn't have our own rooms growing up. We were poor enough so that a curtained partition in the living room served as our makeshift wall. So, one can understand on that superficial level why my mother couldn't just send me to my room. Economics didn't allow it. But neither did the enormity of my crime—dishonoring my mother—allow it. Instead my mother sent me to *her* room, her mother's room, her grandmother's room, her great-grandmother's room. How could I act as I did knowing from what traditions, what roots, what culture I had sprung? How could I desecrate when I had no right to? And upon my return to the States—whether it was days later or years later—I had to ask myself these questions: And if I still want to fit in, how has the need to do so transformed? How has my newly acquired self-understanding and self-respect altered the way that I choose to fit in? Once I acknowledged that by dishonoring my mother I dishonored myself and my culture, I accepted and understood the reasoning that went behind such an extravagant punishment. If at twelve years old I could not comprehend the gravity of my crime against my mother, I could at least extrapolate, from the gravity of my punishment, that I had finally done the abominable. I needed that—to know that I could actually be held accountable, to know that I was wrong. I needed to know that my insult to her merited retribution and maybe even wrath. But above all, I needed to know that at least this much was true—that I was not "*san manman*," either literally or figuratively.

🌹 RETURN

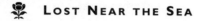 ## LOST NEAR THE SEA

Leslie Chassagne

I came here to find you again
to walk where you walked,
to see if you outlived the house
with the broken planks,
that beach house that once let in
fingers of moonlight, giving wasps
their final dance

I came here to find you again
to stand on a jagged rock
waiting for the light of each wave
to be sucked into the sand
the distant tattoos of the trees
to be scraped by the glowing armor
of the clouds and the majestic and tender palms

I came here to find you again
there have been nights when I have slept soundly
but still I hear you
yelling waist deep in the sea

191

"throw me the mask, there's a shadow there
quickly, quickly," not wanting to miss
any life in the water
Now the sea is turning your ghost into a blue
      crab
a hunter who looks for things
that curl up and die in the sand
and I too am now looking for your ghost
near the sea

I came here to find you again
you wearing the blue plate of the sky
Your voice is a sword under my bed
with our stories etched on the blade,
stories told in your *dossu-marassa* voice
a voice that stutters
with the maleficent jingle of exile

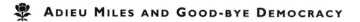

ADIEU MILES AND GOOD-BYE DEMOCRACY

Patrick Sylvain

Prior to mid September 1991, I can honestly say I was a happy man. I was twenty-five years old, an activist, a teacher living in Avon, Massachusetts, a recently married poet, and my son, Kamil, was soon to celebrate his first birthday. In addition to all of this personal bliss, it was the first time in the history of my country that a democratic government, led by a popular nonconformist priest named Jean-Bertrand Aristide, had been elected.

Unfortunately, my own exhilaration and Haiti's jubilee was only to be a temporary affair. On September 29, 1991, I was heading to Cambridge, Massachusetts, to do a poetry reading when all of a sudden, a solemn voice from National Public Radio came through my car radio announcing the death of my favorite trumpeter, Miles Davis. I immediately pulled over and rested my head on the steering wheel, having flashes of my father, reminding me that Miles had spent some time in Haiti. Before long, my body started shaking and I knew that something else was about to go wrong. I found myself crying as I drove toward Harvard Square to visit a friend before my reading.

Soochi was a young Chinese-American woman who was finishing her B.A. at Harvard. She and I often spent hours discussing philosophy, literature, and music. That Saturday evening, she was working at one of the Harvard offices, and I needed her cheerfulness before doing the reading.

As soon as I arrived in her office, she asked me in the softest, gentlest voice, "Have you heard?"

"Yes," I said.

She walked up to me and embraced me as if to say that everything was going to be all right. The way she hugged me was not sexual, but it was the first time that we had held on to one another in that fashion. Abruptly, the image of my wife came rushing through my head. I asked Soochi if I could use her phone to call home.

When my wife answered the phone, I informed her of Miles's passing and told her that given the circumstances, I felt heavy-hearted about the reading.

"Why don't you come home?" said my wife. "I don't know why you sacrifice yourself so much for those things; you are not even getting paid. By the way, a certain Yvon called, he said it was urgent. Listen, we miss you. Come home soon."

After I got off the phone, Soochi offered me a cup of hot chocolate and suggested that I write down my immediate thoughts on Miles. She slipped Miles's CD, *So What?* on the office CD player and walked out of the room. Inhaling the hot chocolate aroma, I wrote what became the last five lines of my poem "Adieu Miles."

> I stumble onto a key
> and the man with the horn
> turns his back
> and walks away
> his trumpet blows tears.

When Soochi came back into the office, she sat down next to me to read what I had written. She effortlessly kissed my left eye and then my forehead. I knew that I was crying again when I tasted my own tears.

I moved away from Soochi to return my friend Yvon's call.

"It's going to happen for real now," Yvon said. "There's going to be a coup in Haiti."

I excused myself and thanked Soochi for her kindness. Outside, I sat in my car for a minute and wept some more. I felt like I was buried in a barrel of hot molasses. After more than two hundred years of struggle, Haiti was heading for further disaster and there was nothing anyone could do about it. It was as if we had a preordained rendezvous with Lucifer.

I had been in Haiti only a few weeks before, for the two-hundredth anniversary of Bois Caiman, the 1791 *Vodou* ceremony that had launched the Haitian revolution. With Aristide's election still recent, my fellow countrymen had seemed extremely joyful, almost intoxicated with happiness. In retrospect, I thought, maybe the country had been too consumed with euphoria and had forgotten about the constant menace of our military coups.

During the Bois Caiman commemoration festivities on the lawn of the national palace in Port-au-Prince, a few tipsy soldiers had vowed that there would never be another coup d'état in Haiti. Gladdened by their resolve, I had embraced them in camaraderie, feeling reassured that they had absorbed the spirit of revolution that rang over Bois Caiman that night long ago, when slaves had dreamt of creating a nation, vowing to always live freely in it or die fighting for it.

Later that same night, with the soldiers' voices still ringing in my head, I had met with Manno Charlemagne, a Haitian singer and activist who had achieved national-hero status in Haiti due to his protest songs. Manno, a friend and mentor, sang against the rule of the *tonton macoutes* in Haiti and the meddling of the United States in our national affairs. That night, Manno told me that he knew that then Vice President Dan Quayle had been meeting with high-ranking Haitian military officers and that since the American government—particularly the Central Intelligence Agency—was unhappy with Jean-Bertrand Aristide, a coup was in the making.

In spite of Manno's warning, I decided to indulge in the pleasures that my country could still offer: beach parties, jet skiing, nightfall skinny-dipping. The next Saturday, just before sunset, I—along with eight friends and family members whom I had not seen in ten years of voluntary exile—rented a small boat and rowed south towards Le Lambi while feasting on baked lobsters, conch, and homemade liqueurs. We sang, joked, and laughed as though it were our last night on earth. On the shore, some of our poorer compatriots cursed at us while others sang along and laughed at the jokes that our loud voices carried across the water.

When we docked in Le Lambi, we spotted a group of men lounging on the beach with prostitutes. At one point, Roland, one of my friends, recognized someone I had grown up with as a child in Haiti and shouted to him, "Hey Jean, tonight is your last night to have sex before the coup."

On the way back, every time we passed by a group of people, we loudly announced to them that there might be a military coup that night. Even though I was laughing, it still disturbed me that we had become a culture so accustomed to military coups that they could so easily become the subject of sad jokes.

When I returned home to the United States, my wife had wanted to know how the country was and how it seemed like the future was going to be. Her memory of Haiti was very limited. She had left there for Belgium when she was eight years old and a few years later had moved to Massachusetts, where we had met almost two years before.

The night of my return, I put our son to bed sensing a silent tension between us. My wife didn't like that I was gone so much, leaving her alone, however briefly, with our infant son. Besides, she thought Haiti was now a dangerous place, where I could have gotten hurt or killed.

To avoid an argument, I kissed my wife and son good-night and went to my office in our house cellar to drown all life's uncertainties in Miles's music until I fell asleep.

My wife's unhappiness about the trip did not last very long. Soon we were once again telling each other jokes and flirting as though we were still courting. And of course our son was always there to increase our delight.

Two days before the coup was to happen, however, on September 27, I received a phone call from a friend of mine, a key political player in Haiti, who informed me that the wheels were now in motion to unseat President Aristide. My friend requested that I alert the members of the Boston Lavalas Committee, a pro-Aristide coalition, that something big was about to happen.

After that phone call, my wife expressed her concern that I was going to be consumed by long political meetings, protests, and demonstrations that would take away from my time with her and our son. Even though she was concerned about Haiti's future, it was our marriage and our family that she wanted to protect and save. That night, after countless hours on the phone, I was assured by friends in Haiti that the coup had been stopped even before it could happen, the situation was under control, Aristide and the people had maintained power. As soon as my wife realized that things had returned to normal in Haiti, she became more affectionate toward me. It looked as though I would be staying home with our family, not out protesting the abrupt end of a fragile new democracy.

The following day, after work, I picked up my son from the

house of my mother, who was kind enough to look after him while my wife and I worked. Once at home, I fed my son and put him in his chair, then started on a special dinner for my wife. I stewed some lobsters in a special rum-raisin sauce I had concocted, baked some sweet potatoes, then boiled some corn on the cob.

When my wife walked into the house, she was taken by surprise. The living room and the kitchen were lit with vanilla-scented candles, and the sensuous melodies of Miles's "Porgy and Bess" resounded within the walls. Speechless, my wife smiled from ear to ear, hugging both me and our son.

Unfortunately, we would never be that happy again. On the twenty-ninth, Miles died, and on the thirtieth the military coup in Haiti finally took place. I was devastated. During the first week of the coup alone, the Haitian military murdered eight hundred people. My friends at the Boston Lavalas Committee and I began organizing and participating in marches and demonstrations in front of key governmental buildings in Boston as well as in front of the United Nations Headquarters in New York and the White House in Washington, D.C. A week into the coup, I was spending more time traveling and in meetings than I ever had in my married life. My wife did not like it and so our marital quarrels became more common and it took much longer for us to reconcile.

Two weeks after our son's birthday and roughly a month after Miles's death and the coup, my wife suggested that we separate. More than feeling sad and guilty for having imposed my political activities on our marriage, I felt horrible about the idea of no longer being close to my son, or being unable to see his gradual growth over the years. I knew that I was a good father and was constantly striving to become a better one, for which my wife had praised me. However, I could not stand by and watch what was happening to my country and remain apolitical and silent. If only my wife had been more supportive, I told myself, perhaps our marriage would have been saved.

When I realized she was serious about me vacating the house, I thought, rather than completely giving up on the marriage, it would be better to stay away for a couple of days in order to rethink all that was happening. I was in a state of shock. It was as if I were holding a handful of sand and watching each grain slip from my grasp.

One Friday afternoon, after my wife and I had been apart for awhile, I found myself at the Magazine Street Beach on the left bank of the Charles River in Cambridge, watching the ducks on the dock seek shelter before sunset. I sat on a three-by-four-foot rock that once served as a boat anchor as a few kayakers loaded their kayaks on top of their cars. The wind turned from brisk to chill as it got dark. I sat there with my eyes closed and listened to waves rolling onto the shore. I felt like those ducks, seeking shelter in the fleeting glory of a sunset that would never be again. To my surprise, Soochi walked up from behind me and placed her hands on my shoulders. She offered me Miles's last recorded CD, *Doo-Bop*.

In 1994, after three years in exile in the United States, Aristide was finally able to return and resume his presidency in Haiti. During his exile, I went through a painful divorce and custody battle that nearly bankrupted both my wife and myself. I soothed my own unhappiness and personal pain by becoming even more deeply involved in political meetings, marches, by reading and writing my poetry with a fervor that I believed would someday contribute to saving my country.

After Aristide's return, with more time to ponder all that had taken place, I had to finally admit to myself that perhaps one's country, one's idealism and dreams should not take precedent over one's life. My marriage, like most people's, had not been perfect; however, my political activities had certainly accelerated our separation and eventual divorce. Many of the men I have attended political meetings with and have been at demonstrations with have spent countless hours in court, or in counseling trying to salvage their marriages or attain visitation rights to see their children.

As sorrowful as this is, I still ask myself whether our sacrifices have really contributed to any permanent changes for Haiti. Frankly, I am not sure. Can we say that all women in Haiti are safe because we no longer have wives? Can we say that every Haitian child will grow up happy, well-fed, and educated because we can now only see our sons and daughters on alternate weekends? I have spent many days and nights crying over the fact that I can now see my only child, my beloved son, at the end of the week.

I wish I could say, like Miles, that my political and personal life has been one of "few regrets and little guilt." But that would not be the case. If anything it is full of regrets and a lot of guilt. But only about that particular period in my life. These days, though I must redefine my vision of happiness, I am happy. If I were to relive all this again, I would tread with more caution and never for one second lose sight of the fact that more important than anything else, I have a son to be a father to.

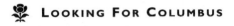 **LOOKING FOR COLUMBUS**

Michel-Rolph Trouillot

I was looking for Columbus, but I knew that he would not be there.
Down by the shore, Port-au-Prince exposed its wounds to the sun;
and Harry Truman Boulevard, once the most beautiful street in
Haiti, was now a patchwork of potholes.

The boulevard was built for the bicentennial celebration of Port-
au-Prince, which Truman helped finance right between his launch-
ing of the North Atlantic Treaty Organization and the start of the
Korean War. Now it looked like a war zone with no memory of
the celebrations of which it had been the center. Only a few of the
statues erected for the occasion remained. Its fountains had dried up
under two Duvaliers. Its palm trees had shrunk as Haiti had itself. I
turned in front of the French Institute, a living monument to the
impact of French culture on the Haitian elites, and drove toward the
U.S. Embassy, a center of power of a different order. Above a moun-
tain of sandbags, a helmeted black G.I. watched nonchalantly as a
crowd of half-naked boys bathed in a puddle left by yesterday's rain.
He had probably come with the occupying forces that helped restore
President Jean-Bertrand Aristide to power in 1994. The story I was
looking for went back nine years earlier.

I drove by.

I stopped the car at a safe distance from the embassy and started a slow walk on the boulevard. On the buildings around the post office, conflicting graffiti asked the U.S. forces both to stay and to go home. I spotted a statue lying behind a fence across the street. A peddling artist stood next to it, selling paintings and crafts. I greeted the man and asked him if he knew where the statue of Christopher Columbus was.

I had vague memories of the statue. I only remembered its existence from my adolescent wanderings. The few images I could summon came from Graham Greene's *The Comedians*. It was under the watchful eye of Columbus that the heroes of that story, later played by Richard Burton and Elizabeth Taylor, consummated their illicit love. But the bust on the grass was no Columbus. The painter confirmed my doubts. "No," he said, "this is a statue of Charlemagne Péralte."

Péralte was the leader of a nationalist army that fought the first occupation of Haiti by the United States in the 1920s. From the pictures the Marines took of him after they had crucified him on a door, I knew he was a thin dark man. The bust on the grass was visibly that of a white male, rather stocky. "You're sure this is Péralte?" I asked again. "Sure this is Péralte," replied the painter. I moved closer and read the inscription. The sculpture was a bust of Harry Truman.

"Where is the Columbus one?" I asked.

"I don't know. I am not from Port-au-Prince," replied the man. "Maybe it is the one that used to be near the water."

I walked to the place he indicated. No statue was there. The pedestal still existed, but the sculpture was missing. Someone had inscribed in the cement: "Charlemagne Péralte Plaza." Truman had become Péralte and Péralte had replaced Columbus.

I stood there for another half hour, asking each passerby if he or she knew what had happened to the Columbus statue. I knew the story: I was in Port-au-Prince when Columbus disappeared. I just wanted confirmation, a test of how public memory works and how history takes shape in a country with the lowest literacy rate on this side of the Atlantic.

I was almost ready to give up when a young man replayed for me the events I had first heard about in 1986. In that year, at the fall of Jean-Claude Duvalier's dictatorship, the most miserable people of Haiti's capital had taken to the streets. They had loosed their anger upon every monument that they associated with the dictatorship. A number of statues had been broken into pieces; others were simply removed from their bases. This was how Truman came to find himself on the grass.

Columbus had a different fate, for reasons still unknown to me. Perhaps the illiterate demonstrators associated his name with colonialism. The mistake, if mistake there was, is understandable: the word *kolon* in Haitian means both Columbus and a colonist. Perhaps they associated him with the ocean from which he came. At any rate, when the angry crowd from the neighboring shanty towns rolled down Harry Truman Boulevard, they seized the statue of Columbus, removed it from its pedestal, and dumped it into the sea.

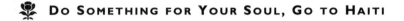

Babette Wainwright

Boarding the van in Port-au-Prince, for the poor southern Haitian village of Jeannette, I intentionally sat separate from the missionaries. This was a humanitarian work mission, not a vacation tour, and I wasn't there to socialize. Instead, I sat next to my friend, Kathy, who had volunteered to provide free dental care to the people in Jeannette for ten days; I was serving as her translator.

Riding in the seat directly behind the driver—a bright young man with many interests and a deep curiosity about life—we spent the time chatting with him in *Kreyòl*. He suggested that we buy the local candy we craved from four vendors at four different stands. "That way, we can help each one make a little money today, instead of giving all the business to just one person." We talked about ways to uplift the country, ways for people to help each other, imagining something like the volunteer systems in the United States.

Kathy and I were going to Jeannette along with the Haiti Mission of the Episcopal Church of Milwaukee, which has been financing a school, church, and mission house in Jeannette for over eleven years. The Mission coordinator had approached me a year before for *Kreyòl* lessons, and had shown me the project's promotional literature, which proclaimed, "Do something for your soul, go to Haiti."

The brochure described yearly "hands on" visits during which visitors could meet and interact with the people of Jeannette and attempt to make a difference in their lives. I decided to go along, paying eleven hundred dollars for a trip back to my homeland. (Although the actual traveling costs were under five hundred dollars, I was told that this trip would be a fund-raiser for the project so I gladly agreed to pay more.)

Our trip from Haiti's capital to Jeannette took four hours. For four hours, the "poorest country in the Western Hemisphere" gave the missionaries, Kathy, and myself its best display of dust, rags, huts, and seaside trash dumps. Kathy wept as we passed a few cadavers of young men in gutters. According to our driver, they were thieves whose bodies no one dared claim, so they were left by the roadside to rot. The members of the Mission seemed unmoved.

At last, we reached the entrance to the small village of Jeannette. Suddenly the missionaries began blowing up balloons and throwing them to a parade of screaming children. The driver shook his head disapprovingly as the children ran dangerously into the road. The missionaries laughed. The scene reminded me of my childhood, watching François "Papa Doc" Duvalier throw pennies out of his limousine window as he rode through the slums of Port-au-Prince. Had I paid so dearly to come to Haiti to contribute to the further dehumanization of my own people?

During our stay in Jeannette, we were lodged in the priest's living quarters, a luxurious mission house equipped with all the amenities: water, modern bathrooms, and comfortable furniture. A garage was under construction. I learned that it had cost eight thousand dollars to build. The priest was a tall, imposing Haitian man in his seventies. He had a long gray beard that made me think of Rasputin. Always lurking behind the missionaries, he seemed to have disdain for them, even while they were in awe of him and his "projects."

The priest's projects for the people of Jeannette included a small
dark church, and two school buildings with tiny dark rooms and
blank walls. The teachers' dormitories resembled jail cells. Ironically,
prior missionaries had once spent an entire trip stenciling the dank
concrete walls of the dormitories "à la Norwegian." A clinic, which
the brochures had advertised as well-stocked, had no bathroom facilities, no running water, and no electricity. I was told that even
the light bulb that lit the clinic during our visit would be removed
by the priest as soon as the missionaries left. I watched as a clinic
helper hauled heavy buckets of water to an unsanitary bathroom
where medical implements were being scrubbed, while hundreds of
patients waited all day to be seen.

Most people in Jeannette must go for days without a proper meal,
walk for miles to fetch water, use the bushes as their bathroom, live
with infected skin wounds if they can't pay the two gourdes or
twelve U.S. cents required to see the nurse in this clinic. Teachers
report that the local children are so hungry that many are unable to
stay alert in class. The teachers themselves often go without food. A
teacher's aide who shares a shack with eight members of his family
told me that he could not afford to replace his torn shoes. In the
meantime, he watched quietly as the eight-thousand-dollar garage
was built to accommodate the Haiti Project's van. People do not
need to build elaborate garages for their cars in Jeannette, especially
when their homes are fenced in. Leaving the car in the yard or under
a simple carport would offer it plenty of protection. With the eight
thousand dollars for this garage, the project could have built over a
dozen solid homes, or an open-air cafeteria to provide a balanced
midday meal for all the students and school personnel, five days a
week, for a year.

In addition to obvious wastefulness, the missionaries also showed
a lack of sensitivity toward the people of Jeannette. In one instance,

the Haiti Project leaders kept the cook waiting long past her working hours and then, while indulging in one of their nightly cocktail parties, declared that, "All she had wanted was to go and party."

A young Haitian woman who had spent an entire morning helping us in the clinic was invited by the nurse to join us for lunch. This gesture displeased the church members, who rushed to take the food away, sending the young woman running from the table in shame. I talked with a man who had designed a number of greeting cards and embroidered several items of clothing hoping that the mission would use them for fund-raising. Project members ignored him, patronizing instead an art shop in Port-au-Prince that was a well-known sweat shop.

If in fact the goal was to develop self-reliance in Jeannette, not only would the missionaries have supported local entrepreneurs, but during the yearly "hands-on" trips the missionaries also would have brought with them appropriate items such as farming tools, fabrics, blankets, lamps, and up-to-date medical supplies, rather than the hard candy, plastic cups, balloons, and sample vials of expired medicines. These items did nothing to help poor people escape their oppression and misery. Furthermore, they contributed to the significant amount of dumping I saw around the clinic and the school yard.

Since none of the missionaries on this particular trip had bothered to master the language of the people they served, I wondered if they could assess the people's needs and measure the effectiveness of their interventions. For example, What happened to the young people once they completed the last grade at their Mission school? They returned to their shacks to face hunger with the rest of the community.

I saw and heard discontented people who watched as the priest obtained a TV antenna, solar and wind generators, a garage, and a bamboo fence to keep them out of the mission house, while their children remained malnourished and thirsty in the mud huts. Weren't the people of Jeannette the reason so much money was donated to this project? Weren't their pathetic photographs used to touch the donors' hearts and pockets?

Now it is clear to me what the promotional bulletin meant when it said: "Do something for your soul, go to Haiti." For this mission, Haiti is a place to relax, have nightly cocktail parties, and feel important as you watch the natives beg for your leftovers and trash. Returning to my homeland with the Haiti Mission project did do something for my soul: It wounded it deeply.

🌷 A POEM ABOUT WHY I CAN'T WAIT
GOING HOME AGAIN AND AGAIN AND AGAIN

Gina Ulysse

Every morning from the time I was three
I had to open my mouth to receive
two tablespoons full of emulsion scott
sometimes I would pinch my nose so I couldn't smell it
making it easier to swallow that pasty white liquid
that left my tongue tasting of salty tears and cod liver oil
Often we had to chase it with homemade V-8
watercress celery beets spinach carrots and all sorts of
other things that grow in the earth to give little weaklings strength

Despite the grimaces pouts tears
despite the nos the I don't want tos the cries the wails
the screams that often preceded this ritual
eventually I would drink it
not because it's good for me
but because I had to I didn't have a choice
I had to open my mouth
let it slime down my throat
and swallow

When I was about fifteen
One day my father called all three of us in the living room
and told us we had to let go of our dreams
and be serious about the future
Poor man not even a son to carry on his name
he had been cursed with three girls
and we wanted to be a singer a dancer and a writer
After calling us by our names he said
I want a doctor a lawyer and a dentist
I remember saying to him
I don't care if I never have any money
(though I would change my mind later)
I don't care if I never have any money
even if I live in a tent as long as I have my music
What are you asking me that I live this life my life for you
In all my sassiness I dared him.
And when would I live my life? when you die?
the horror on his face I have since forgotten
but I remember mother verbally mourning her wasted life
having given him the best years of her life
and realizing that I only get to do this "life thing" once
so I was going to do it on my terms
as long as I have a choice

I remember the first time I went back to Haiti
It had been 17 years
but I had to hide in a hotel so daddy wouldn't know I was there
Desperate to refill all the gaps in my past
I stole back memories at night to retrace my childhood
I begged my cousin to drive me around
to the house on rue darguin

but it was long gone
and had been replaced with an edifice that
breathed the same coldness as the Pentagon
then we went to the gingerbread house
that too had been demolished and reconstructed
though the mango tree was still there
le petit chaperon rouge had been closed for years
vines interlaced with the iron of the gate

I went back again two years later
and I remember a conversation with a man
who has lived in Haiti longer than I did
this white man who says he loves my country
the country that I saw in newspapers and on TV
for seventeen years
the country that for the longest time I only went to in translation
we were talking about class and color
I was asserting my gramscian ideals
about the importance of and the need to fight both wars—
the war of maneuver and the war of position
especially the war of position
so we can take back spaces
hence why I tie my head with a scarf when I go to those places
you think they care he replied
they don't care about your aunt jemima head
uhmm! even after over twenty years in this country
you still have no other references I said quietly
Oh these ethnic notions I thought enraged
after over twenty years in my country his social limits were intact
for me that was the end of the conversation
after all this was not a teach-in

**How do you overturn four hundred years of history
in less than one century?**

I've been thinking a lot about writing a poem
about the meaning of the word *diplomacy*
about how this word is just another four letter word
about how this word is just another way to say
I am going to fuck you
not only are you not going to enjoy it
but when I am done with you
you're sure to say thank you
and like my sistahgurl says you might even pay me for it
in accrued debt interest

Can life exist without ideals
Can life exist without dreams

                    where does your soul go
                    when all you do is function
                    where does your spirit go
                    when all you do is function

I am only 31 years old and I am getting so cynical
I am trying not to be
I've been reading Shakti Gawain
trying to do creative visualization
trying to imagine

                              <imagine all the people
                              living life in peace>

trying to imagine a better world
so I can change my world
so I can change the world

But I have been having a lot of difficulty
I keep remembering my friend B with her three kids
who after a year still can't get a job
its not because she's not qualified
or that she's not trying
but because she's not from the right family
she doesn't have the right connections
and her skin is too damn dark
worse
she doesn't play by the rules of the game
she doesn't do safe cocktail conversations
she was on the sidewalks in the 80s
bringing down the second revolution
she was there on the streets
in front of the palace
in front of ministries
in front of police stations
waiting
waiting to lay claim to dead bodies
no one else would acknowledge for fear of losing their lives
you know in Haiti one often inherits social scars by association
you know in Haiti one often inherits fatal scars by association
scars
wars
social fatal
death by association
tell me how to imagine a better world in this place
tell me how to imagine a better world in this place
       where even after operation restore democracy
       that came bounded with IMF loans
       International Mother Fucking loans
       for the structurally adjusted

where the rules of the game are
I am going to fuck you
and you are not going to enjoy it
tell me how do you imagine a better world in this place
tell me how to imagine a better world in this place
where the rules of the game is this diplomacy
where blackness still equals poverty
where even after over 400 years
still too black too strong not French enough
never really French enough
and the new generations don't want to be men

raging youths are now more committed
to seeing blood run
raging youths are now more committed
to seeing blood run
to seeing blood run on sidewalks
just to see blood run through the streets
next to expensive cars
outside of élite-owned stores
because they say they have had enough
                    jan l pase l pase
                    jan l mouri l mouri
                    however it goes down it goes down
                    however it dies it dies
the end result is still the same
the revolution is not over
                         <Call Mr. Martin
                         tell him to build a coffin>
the revolution is not over they cry as they die

they have had too much adversity
this is the generational gap
don't need to ask them when are they going to grow up
when are they going to grow out of this phase
it is not a phase this is about the game
it was at the university that they learned the rules
through liberation theology they learned they were comrades
it was at the university that they learned
the multiple meanings of the word *diplomacy*
how you have to be pliable
acquiescent
don't make waves you don't get the perks
no gains if you misbehave like a good little *nèg*
that's what you are being trained to be
a docile body without integrity
like the ancestor who sold my ancestor to the west
depi nan ginen nèg pat vle wè nèg

> *gede nibo gad sa vivan yo fè mwen*
> *plante mayi m mayi m tounen rozo*
> *rozo tounen banbou*
> *banbou tounen ponya*
> *ponya yo ponyade m gede*

**How do you overturn four hundred years of history
   in less than one century?**

And I keep thinking back to my life here
And I keep thinking back to my life right here
in this white power center
ain't no misbehavin' here

in the ivory tower
abounded with liberals and marxist scholars
where liberalism is rhetorically defined
as a floating signifier associated with
the ever-growing pony tail
the peace sign
the old leather jacket from undergrad
the backwards baseball cap
nightly homage to the celestial herb to justify being a function
commitments
commitment to the metaphysics of diversity
commitments
to the environment to animal rights
the pet projects
and pet cultures
signifying signifiers
are recreating structures
these signifying signifiers are recreating structures
these signifying signifiers are recreating bourgeois structures

bourgeois bourgeoisie bougi bouginess
blackness bouginess blackness
contradictions
disjunctures
                         underplayed identities
                         downpressing privilege
down
         down
down you got to keep it down
sometimes it just wants to rise up
but you gotta keep it down

Shut your mouth!!!!
stuff it in your mouth
just keep your mouth shut and get out
ram it down your throat
deep down your throat
swallow
it
down
you're being forced
to
deep throat
But I don't want to
I don't want to
swallow
it
down
you gotta keep it down
you gotta keep it down
why you have to be down to keep it real
      downplaying privilege
little white rebels wanna be niggers
and niggers wanna be niggaz
bourgeois blues
opportunities denied
blackness bouginess
disjunctures?
contradictions?

In Haiti the bourgeoisie funded coups
in Jamaica uptown bougies tried to silence a revolution

but rastafari had a free black mind
so they self-fashioned an everyday resistance
the self-fashioning of an everyday SEXIST resistance
                   an everyday HOMOPHOBIC resistance
                                 <don't let them fool ya
                                 or even try to school ya>

blackness bouginess blackness
in the Caribbean bouginess has funded revolutions
little white rebels wanna be niggers
and rebelling niggers wanna be niggaz
these signifying signifiers are just recreating bourgeois structures

Can life exist without ideals
Can life exists without dreams
                   where does your soul go
                       when all you do is function
                   where does your spirit go
                       when all you do is function

Lately I have been thinking a lot about writing
a poem about class comfort
and color and privilege and guilt
about the social luxury of whiteness
about the social luxury of the white skin
a poem about the rules of the game
and I think back to the keeping it real conference
how we had the rhetoric to deconstruct performance
the performance of blackness and black identities
but we couldn't talk about black privilege
for fear of having to talk about black guilt

like the good doctor says we can't talk
about the fact that we like trashing on the weak
because we don't have the courage to confront the powerful
in this place
in this white power center
this bastion of liberalism
where ANTHROPOLOGY incubates racism
where anthropology INCUBATES racism
where anthropology incubates RACISM
this place of learning who the players are
what the rules of the game are
and how to play and win

> How do you play knowing that at every moment
> in time your identity is in question
> How do you win when at every moment
> in time your identity is in question

I'm criminal
compulsive alertness
always having to be alert
criminal
always ready to answer questions
that never get asked
because of assumptions
that lead to even more questions

> \<All I need is a good defense
> coz I'm feeling like a criminal\>

How do you overturn four hundred years of history
in less than one century?

Since this is about why I can't wait
I am gonna tell you why I am so tired

why I'm so tired
of not being able to imagine a better world
so I can change my world so we can change the world
why can't we talk about the things that make you wanna
can't talk about the things that make you wanna holler
make me wanna scream
cry
yell
let my people go
let my people go
right here
right now
right here
let me go
how far will we go
when we're still in chains
I can't wait because I am tired
tired of smiling
tired of masking
I'm tired of signifyin'
tired of being on the front line
tired of fighting the same damned isms
daily
I am tired of wearing this suit of steel
I am tired of being weighed down by armor
I am tired of carrying a banner of love
while THE war
still rages
on

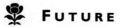 **FUTURE**

❀ LAZARUS RISING: AN OPEN LETTER TO MY DAUGHTER

Myriam J. A. Chancy

Ma très chère Aimée,

You have not yet even arrived and already I worry about what your life may be like, far from Haitian shores. I can already see it— the day you enter kindergarten, all frills and curls, bright-eyed, with some butterflies making your little stomach queasy: No one will know how to pronounce your name. Aimée, like the pan-Africanist Martinican writer Aimé Césaire, but named for love. Aimée: French for beloved. Will you know to tell your teachers and schoolmates how to pronounce it correctly? They will insist on transforming it into "Amy." Will you wince, misrecognize yourself, crawl into your infantile shell and reemerge as something closer to their expectations as I had done so many years ago only to return, at long last, to my own bright self, name and all? I must pause now and smile at the thought of how long you have been loved and awaited. You are bound to arrive in the next century, not so long from now. I want this letter to be a bridge for you, to people and events already come to pass that you will not have the opportunity to experience, but which are nonetheless yours to hold and have, a part of your heritage.

Our lives may intersect in two different planes, you in the flowering of a new life, me in the wilting of an aging one. I write you this, then, so you will know your mother before she was your mother, when she was young, full of life and dreams—dreaming still about the day you would be in her midst. I want to try and set down some details of what life has been like for me as a displaced Haitian woman, growing up in lands not my own, in places that have demanded my integration and assimilation, a betrayal of my Haitianness and the various heritages that make up that identity; I want you to know some of these things in case you must repeat those lessons and I am not there to speak to, or, in case I become (between now and the moment of your arrival) the kind of adult who no longer knows how to listen to the wisdom of children's voices, who no longer daydreams or draws boxes on scribbling paper with elephants inside, invisible to the naked eye. I write these things to you so that you may know and understand that you are not alone in the things you will experience. You will not be the first and you will certainly not be the last.

RACE LESSONS

I want to begin, briefly, with the story of my family's movements back and forth between Port-au-Prince and North America. From the moment of my birth in 1970 until the age of five, the four of us shuttled back and forth from Haiti to Quebec. At one point, as my parents sought to establish themselves in North America, my brother and I, ages three and one respectively, lived either with an aunt or our grandmother for over a year's time. For this reason, I did not realize until we moved to English Canada in 1975 and I attended school there that we no longer lived permanently in Haiti. Prior to the age of five, after a few months on the continent, I had felt that we would return to Haiti and, eventually, we always did return. Haiti was home: There we were surrounded by family members of all ages. We went to school and had schoolmates. When we returned to Canada, it was the absence of the rest of our family, the smiling aunts and uncles, our grandparents, which weighed heavily upon my child's heart.

All of my childhood, even after the returns to Haiti came to an end at the age of eight, the memories of my birthplace remained the strongest. Those memories have molded my spirit, a certainty I have of what it means to be Haitian; of what it means to me to have been born in a place where I was welcomed by many open arms, into the bosom of a large family that has since become dispersed and fragmented; of what it means to be born in a place where, despite poverty, caste, and colorism, to be of African descent or mixed heritage, to know one's heritage is as important as knowing the names of your grandmothers, as important as remembering the source of your own naming.

Yes, Haiti continues to be afflicted by various problems—social, political, economic. Before the droughts that plagued Eastern Africa occurred in the mid-eighties and caused widespread famine, Haiti was categorized as the poorest country in the world. It is now the poorest country in the Western Hemisphere. It was also the first black republic in this hemisphere. Yet, while Haiti is often lauded for the triumph of the slave revolt that defeated Napoleon Bonaparte's troops and culminated in independence in 1804, her people are consistently denigrated and forced to endure economic blockades and racialized global trade practices that unduly penalize Haiti precisely because of its early triumph over European imperialism. Still, even diminished, we remain the same prideful people who kept our traditions well-enough alive to organize ourselves and successfully resist enslavement. Despite syncretism and outside influences, Africa remains in our veins as well as in the weathered features of our faces, rainbow hues, Arawak cheekbones, and all textures of hair known to man.

Coming from such a background, transplanted into a Euro-dominated culture, it was a shock then, to find out that the white faces that looked into mine when I was a child were, indeed, white. I assumed, then, that everyone of a lighter hue was a person of color because I had been born to a Haitian mother who, throughout my Canadian childhood, was often taken for white. It was a shock to learn that, in Canada (as in the United States), there is a clear line drawn between those who are of color and those who are considered not to be. It was a shock to be turned away from the next door neighbor's house at age four, to be told by her mother that I could not play with my friend inside her house. The same woman told me later that summer, as she was bronzing herself in the sun, that she wanted to be dark like me. Dark like me? I wondered how she could both envy and loathe me. I thought she was a silly woman then, not understanding that I had had my first encounter with racism. It was in Winnipeg, a prairie city in the middle of the country, that I was to find out categorically what it meant to be black in a country not your own. I was not even ten years old when walking down the street, I could hear young white men muttering under their breaths as they walked by, "Nigger." It was a matter of color and it was a matter of pride. How dare a young, brown woman walk down the street and hold up her head high, and smile, and look people in the eye? This is what I did, not knowing I was meant to look down and away and step aside. Not looking away, however, brought me something else I had not expected, the affirmations of other people of color, especially those who were Native American, Indian, or Arab, who often mistook me for one of their own because of my mixed-race features blending African, Arawak, French, and Spanish lineages. Still, general invisibility—social, political, economic—has a way of putting a brown person in her place, no matter how high she holds her head up, how brilliant her smile, no matter how sure her step down a crowded street or way. These were my Canadian lessons. Yet something in me refused to assimilate.

Even as I learned to speak perfect, standard English at the age of ten, shedding my French accent, I remained Haitian to the core, prideful. I found myself isolated in my refusal to blend in, isolated by my knowledge of what colonialism had done to enslaved Africans dispersed throughout the so-called New World, and isolated by my fervent desire to make that knowledge count.

It is this isolation, Aimée, that I most hope you will not have to relive. It is, in a way, an immigrant legacy. I came into the world as one Duvalier regime neared its end and another was just about to begin. At that time, outside (as inside) of Haiti, one had to be careful of who one got close to: It was clear that foreigners were not to be trusted (who knew who might turn a racist eye toward you or when?). Haitians outside of one's immediate family were also suspect (for who knew when something you might say might be said to the wrong person, an ear of the government or some *macoutes* who could harm you or your family still left behind?). We lived, therefore, in what was initially a chosen isolation in Quebec City prior to 1975, always being careful who was brought close to the family. After 1975 and our move to English Canada, our social isolation was compounded by a language barrier: Initially, we spoke no English. The cocoon in which we lived then had many layers, both cultural and linguistic; isolation became imposed rather than chosen.

Immigration created a shyness in me that was not natural, and I continue to struggle with it to this day. Since my spirit had remained attached to Haiti, and especially to my maternal grandmother, Alice Limousin, my father's stepmother, I knew without being told directly that there were things happening in Haiti that I was being spared. I remember being warned to be careful of what I said on the phone when speaking to relatives in Haiti: The wires could be tapped. I remember an uncle disappearing one day and the phone calls going back and forth between members of the large family network as we prayed that he would be released from Duvalier's jails. We heard about killings and tortures, and I had nightmares that even as far away as Canada, members of Duvalier's secret police could find me just for thinking the wrong thing. Life was like walking on eggshells. Going home was not an option. Neither was assimilating. I had to create a new reality, one that belonged neither to the new world I had been forced to enter nor to my parents' generation. I began to belong to what I often think of as the lost generation: I identified most clearly with cousins some twenty years older than myself who had been there the day I was born, who had grown up in Haiti before leaving the country (those who could) to seek their fortunes elsewhere. Like them, I could not deny my Haitianness, would not take U.S. citizenship even when I, too, eventually migrated, alone, south of the Canadian border (I had become a Canadian citizen at age five). I regarded my Canadian citizenship for what it was, a passport that allowed me to return to Haiti when I wanted, without hassles; it guaranteed my freedom and allowed me to still belong somewhere, even if that somewhere was not home. Canada did not demand that I strip myself of my identity to remain on her shores as I believe America does. And so I remain a part of a generation born in Haiti during the Duvalier years privy to the memories of parents who had been born in the 1930s, long before that regime dawned, and to those grandparents born before and during the turn of the century. This familial memory has given me a safety net when I fear being overwhelmed by an isolation too unfamiliar to be shared by those around me.

I will be thirty this year, but those in my family with whom I best connect are in their forties and fifties. Because of this intergenerational bonding, I feel as if I have eyes at the back of my head: I stand not between two cultures, one Haitian, the other American, but between generations, one belonging to the pre-Duvalier era and the other belonging to the post-Duvalier era. Sometimes it is like standing in a barren no-man's land, but I know that some of us need to be the in-betweens so the gaps will not bleed, so that the discarded will be remembered and the wounds of forgetfulness staunched.

This year also marks a turning point in my life for I have now reached the age of my mother's orphaning. Perhaps this is also one of the reasons I feel compelled to write this letter, Aimée, because I am aware of living on borrowed time, that every opportunity I have to have a disagreement or a moment of understanding with my own mother is a blessing that ended for her in her twenty-ninth year. She had lost her father earlier at age seven. When she was twenty-nine, her mother passed away. Her loss has led me to think deeply about my own relationship to my mother, to her mother, and to you. What survives? What is forever lost?

When I was eight years old, I met my father's grandmother, my great-grandmother. I remember it as the first time we met though this cannot be possible. The woman I met when I was eight years old was nearing a hundred years of age, small-boned, frail. Yet she saw clearly and spoke a *Kreyòl* that seemed to me to be unlike that of my parents; it contained more of Africa in it, more of the rural in it. Because of this, we could hardly communicate; I was afraid of her too, not because she could do me harm physically, but because I could feel her strong spiritual presence. I remember that she had a *kenèp* tree in her front yard, full of the small, green-shelled fruit that became (and remains) my favorite fruit of all. She encouraged my brother and me to grasp handfuls from the old branches and to eat them on the spot. That afternoon, she also gave us *dous* to eat, a homemade square confection that resembles fudge. I dream of the taste of it sometimes; I have never tasted anything like it since. When she passed away a few years later, the recipe died with her. Now that I am older, always trying to understand better the history and cultural legacy of this place I call home but can only visit from time to time, I think of the conversations we might have had, of the version of *Kreyòl* she spoke that she could have taught me. Although her birth certificate has been lost, she must have been born in the late 1880s, not even a century after the Haitian Revolution. What could she have told us about her childhood memories, of life then? So, you see Aimée, much has already been lost. Like her, but some hundred years after her birth, I am witnessing a century come to a close and I will live the bulk of my life in the next. With this writing, I hope to leave you something for your own days of wonder; something, perhaps, to answer the questions I hope you will have.

EPIPHANY

As I write to you today, resting next to me is a packet of letters my mother gave to me a year or so ago. Some of the letters are written in her mother's hand. This is all I have by which to know her. They are the last letters penned by her my mother received. My mother had just left Haiti for graduate law study in Paris. Her mother intended to visit her there—it would be her own first journey off of the island. The letter paper is thin, the ink beginning to fade in places. The first letter, dated December 1, 1961, begins:

> *Les chants de Noël avaient commencé a me jeter dans l'angoisse; tu sais ce n'est pas du sentiment—quand on les entonne ils me vont droit*

au coeur et me donnent un frisson de coeur qui agit sur tous mes membres est-ce pourquoi je ferai tous mes efforts pour réaliser mon voyage. Il parait que ce sera là ma guérison aussi j'ai commencé sens m'illusioner a confectionner mes linges; il est encore tôt mais cela vaut mieux.

[The Christmas carols had begun to throw me into a deep state of anguish; you know, it isn't nostalgia that I feel, when they are sung they go straight to my heart and send a chill through it that permeates all of my limbs. Thus, I have decided to do all in my power to bring about my voyage; it seems that it will be my cure and so I have begun, without giving in to disillusionment, to make my travel clothes; it is still early for such things, but it is preferable to do so.]

I read these lines and feel the deep emotions my grandmother must have felt at being separated from her youngest daughter. I see in her words also the heart of a poet. I see myself in these lines, knowing how sensitive I am to change of any kind, how deeply loyal to those I love, always missing those who are at a distance. Mama Fofo, as she was called, was an artist of a kind, a seamstress. She was, thus, literally planning to make her clothes for the voyage, in the same loving way that she had made her own daughters' dresses, the same way she had dutifully put fingers to needle, to thread, to cloth in the making of wardrobes for others, back curved over her Singer sewing machine, in order to make a living for herself and her family. She was a single mother raising four children in Haiti from the late 1920s through the 1930s.

Reading Mama Fofo's letters help me to restore some missing links in my own life; they help me to recapture a connection to a woman whom I never met but from whom I have inherited some personality traits: warmth, sensitivity, but also a tendency, at times, not to take best care of myself. Through these letters, I better understand both her and my own character.

Mama Fofo is preparing to go on this voyage which both lifts her spirit and creates great anxiety in her. She does not have the money to go and is trying to call in loans made to friends in need. Many of them refuse to return the money, sums at times as low as twenty dollars. They do not seem to think that the trip is so serious; they do not realize her true need. Mama Fofo's money is lost, so it seems, and in the midst of trying to realize this dream of crossing the Atlantic in order to see her daughter, she finds out that she has placed her trust in the wrong people. She writes: *"réellement on ne doit compter que sur soi"* [really, we can only count on ourselves]. The letters then detail, over the course of a few weeks, what money she has been able to put aside or reclaim. There are gifts from her other children and also from my mother. Mama Fofo was sixty-five at the time she wrote this letter. And I, some thirty years after her death, have just begun to learn such lessons, to be generous without expense to oneself.

I read a meditation today that speaks of this, a Taoist teaching on the theme of caring. It was written by Deng Ming Dao in his book, *365 Tao*. Let me set it down for you here:

Those who follow Tao believe in using sixteen attributes on behalf of others: mercy, gentleness, patience, nonattachment, control, skill, joy, spiritual love, humility, reflection, restfulness, seriousness, effort, controlled emotion, magnanimity, and concentration. Whenever you need to help another, draw upon these qualities. Notice that self-sacrifice is not included in this list. You do not need to destroy yourself to help another. Your overall obligation is to complete your own journey along your personal Tao. As long as you can offer solace to others on your same path, you have done the best that you can.

I believe that Mama Fofo embodied most of the above but it was in the last moments of her life that she realized that she did not need to destroy herself in order to help others. Had she learned this lesson sooner, would she have made it to Paris? Would the last moments of her life have been less fraught with the fear of never seeing her daughter again? Or had she already realized that she was losing a battle against time, losing that battle to her penury, her lesson learned too late?

Her last letter is dated January 4, 1962, three days after Haitian independence is celebrated. Her first lines reveal that she has finally gathered nearly all the money necessary for the voyage. She is missing only eighty-five U.S. dollars. At this point, she hopes that the trip will take place in the coming summer. She writes of possibly selling her house as some businessmen have made her an offer for the property. She hesitates to sell her children's childhood home and is afraid that the affair *"causera ma mort"* [will cause my death]. There are three more letters in the packet, dated the eighth, ninth, and tenth of January 1962. Each recounts the final moments of Mama Fofo, who passed away on Epiphany, the sixth of January 1962, after some days of complaining that her heart was tight as a fist. Did she die of a broken heart? Of a heart attack? This is something only she knew. The letters written by other hands reveal how loved she was by her children and closest family friends, how much love she had during the course of her hard-working life, even though, in the end, she could not make her way to one, among the others, whom she loved greatly.

My mother received Mama Fofo's last letters along with the announcements of her death. How deep her shock, her loss—I cannot imagine. At this age, still reaching out toward my own dreams, I cannot imagine my life without my mother and father even though I see my own parents rarely, living as we do in different countries. I was born eight years after her death, but I am very much like her. My mother and I have had the opportunity to give life to aspects of a relationship that was taken away prematurely, in reverse. I can learn from my grandmother's errors and build on her legacy. Her generosity need not be forgotten. The fact that she passed away on Epiphany, the day on which Catholics celebrate the adoration of the Three Kings bearing gifts for Christ, impresses upon me the necessity of remembering that even within the most humble of beings and across racial, class, and gender lines—there can be a noble heart. It is that heart that I celebrate and want to nurture in myself. It is not lost upon me, too, that Independence Day had just been celebrated and that she could not, as a working-class, single, Haitian woman of a certain age, secure her own independence.

Aimée, when I sense the pain in Mama Fofo's letters, I think that if there is only one thing I can teach you, it would be this: to value and to take the best care of yourself. Without this grounding in your own center of being, the world you are about to enter will be all the more difficult. I have only begun to enact this lesson. It remains my greatest challenge.

RISING

I want to tell you about another Haitian woman, my paternal grandmother, Alice Limousin, whose care for me in my earliest years has left a permanent impression upon my mind, body, and soul. When I began to write you this letter, I reread the last card she wrote me. She was seventy-five years old when she wrote it; she had been

undergoing chemotherapy treatment for advanced breast cancer in
Miami. Because of the absence of preventive health care in Haiti,
her cancer was discovered too late—yet as a member of the working
middle class, she was lucky to have had health attention at all. I had
just begun my first job, fresh out of graduate school, as a college
professor at a private university in the southern United States. I did
not have the time and means to make my way to her side so I wrote
to her instead. She did not reply about her pain. As she always did
in her letters, she thanked me for thinking of her and wrote of her
plans to return to Port-au-Prince for the Christmas holidays. She
missed her home. It is clear from the content of the card that she
knew her days were numbered. She wrote of how much she loved
me. She also wrote advice she had never given me before. A firm
believer in the Catholic Church and its teachings, she counseled me
to stay close to God. Though I left the Catholic Church at the age
of fourteen (objecting to its missionary work in Haiti and other
developing countries, sexist hierarchy, and homophobia), I am a
strong believer in a greater power. I don't know what form that
power takes, but I respect it and I believe I have been able to live
up to the spirit of my grandmother's advice if not to its letter. I have
faith in the energy that surrounds and guides us in this world. On
the back of the card, she tells me that when I need help in the future,
to look to my Bible for assistance. I know she wrote this because
when I was a child and things in my life were beyond my compre-
hension, I would write her a few lines, never letting her know exactly what the problem was, but just that I needed some affirmation.
Months later, often after I had forgotten the source of my earlier
grievance, a letter would appear in response, letting me know that
someone in Haiti held my spirit dear and loved me unconditionally
despite the distance between us. I knew with finality when I read
those lines that she was saying good-bye, just in case, in her own

way. She referred me to the Bible, to John: 11. "There," she wrote, "you can read about everything." I don't know if I turned to that passage then. I don't remember doing so. I may have done so sometime in the haze of the depression that hit me following her death in 1995, three months after I finally had the chance to see her in Haiti, my first trip back to my native land since our family trips had come to an abrupt end in the late seventies. Today, I read this card again, hoping it would provide me with something to pass on to you. And so I turned to John: 11, wondering what was there that could contain the "everything" Mamie (as I have called her from infancy) wrote about. I found, to my surprise, the story of Lazarus and his resurrection from the dead.

This is how the story goes, Aimée: Lazarus, a close friend of Jesus, was very ill. His sisters sent for Jesus to perform a miracle so that Lazarus would not die. Jesus went to him but by the time he reached Lazarus's home, he had already expired. One of Lazarus's sisters tells him: "If you had been here, my brother would not have died." After some discussion, Jesus makes this pronouncement: "I am the resurrection; whoever believes in me, even if he dies, will live; and whoever lives and believes in me will never die." After this they enter the tomb of Lazarus, and find the body already in a state of decay. Jesus calls to Lazarus to walk out of the grave and Lazarus emerges, wrapped in his burial cloth, resurrected.

I read this story and realized what my grandmother had been trying to tell me, in the only words she knew inside and out. She was about to die but she believed in a power greater than herself. She knew she would live in an altered state, somewhere removed from the earth-bound, but still with us. Although I have left the Church and I never thought that I would be recounting a biblical story to you in this way, Aimée, I know that my grandmother was wise to point me in this direction. Because the Bible is, like the

Torah, the Tao Te Ching, the Koran, and so many others, a sacred text. And although my grandmother did not believe in *Vodou*, as I have begun to in my adult years (not firsthand but through extensive reading), this story reminds me of African beliefs in the rebirth of the spirits, the idea that spirits never die. I know that my grand-mother lives on in me and so shall she in you. As long as our memories are alive, so is she and all of the ancestors who preceded her own life. At the end of the card, she expresses concern that I work too hard and live my life alone. She hopes these words will bring me solace in times of loneliness. As I said earlier, though I can't remember if I read the story of Lazarus rising when I received this card or shortly after her death, now, four years later, I am thankful for it as I acknowledge my own rebirth. I am claiming my Haitian-ness in the United States, an identity made especially suspect in this country by racism and xenophobia. I am claiming my solitude and the memories isolation affords me the privilege of revisiting.

Aimée, I am twenty-nine and I have just begun to rise from the ashes of my childhood fears. I was twenty-five when my grand-mother passed away and though I had spent most of those years away from her side (seeing her every three or four years), my body is as if tattooed by the imprints of her palms as she bathed me as a child and fed me baby food as I lay between her bosom and arm. Can any touch be more sacred than this? Much has been made of the fact that the body remembers its injuries, its traumas. But what happens to the good touch, especially when that touch occurs early in life, when a child is full of potential and knows nothing of the difficulties of life? I have been thinking that the body must remember such a touch as sacred, and that if one is blessed with it, whatever traumas the body may sustain later on can be more easily overcome. I believe my body remembers its movements in water as my grandmother bathed me as if they were movements in the womb: safe, soundless, magical. I believe that the first touches we experience in life are as sacred as the last ones, the ones that prepare us for the journey home, to Vilokan, Ginen, Dahomey, or to a glorious heaven. I was not there to bathe her in return, to cleanse the feet that had walked many miles for her children and grandchildren, to close the eyelids that had seen more heartbreak in the busy streets of Port-au-Prince daily than most people in developing countries will experience in a lifetime. After she died, part of my own spirit seemed to follow; I felt as if a limb had been taken away; it ached in the absence of her presence. I have come to understand that it was a necessary loss, one that ensured that I would mature in ways that I had not explored because her presence and memory both provided me with the kind of nurture of soul which discouraged my creation of my own sources of sustenance. I was told at her funeral that the day after I had left Haiti, she took to her bed and never rose from it until her death, as if she had just waited for my return and our last encounter. It is enough for me to know that I was there to embrace her, as she had me, in childhood, in the last months of her life. Now that she is gone, something else has come to be in that space of spiritual connectedness that once belonged to us both—a second chance at life, the opportunity to live out the lessons gleaned from observing my grandmother's existence from a distance: how to be a new kind of Haitian woman, one who reveres the old ways and yet knows her own power and is not afraid of putting that power to good use. I am in the fourth year of my own resurrection and every step forward is small but strong.

The great irony of my life is that it is life in exile which has afforded me the luxury of looking back across time, to appreciate all that is Haiti. Living on the outside has enabled me to learn not only about Haiti but about the rest of the African diaspora. As a woman, there are things I have accomplished that I know both of my grandmothers could not have accomplished in Haiti. No one knows what their dreams might have been, whether one had wanted to be a poet, the other a teacher. They became wives and mothers and their lives were defined by those two words. They sacrificed their personal happiness for their families, never thinking that perhaps they could, by living out those dreams, present them as gifts to their children, especially their female children, as pathways to their own dreams. And yet, it is clear to me that in the strength of their presence in those children's lives, they showed the potential to have accomplished anything they might have set their minds to. They made the most of what they had and this, in itself, makes for a humbling example. Because of their sacrifices, as well as the upheavals in Haiti, I am free in ways that I could not have been there. Yet Haiti remains my compass. How to explain? I think, Aimée, that this, too, will be one of the riddles of your life. But until such time as you may need to consider such a question, I leave you with the parting words of my own grandmother: *"La paix de Dieu soit avec toi"* [May the peace of God be with you]. Whatever gods you may believe in, may they protect you and light your way and may you be a light for others as you have always been to me.

    With love, your mother,

    Myriam Josèphe Aimée Chancy

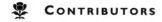 **CONTRIBUTORS**

Edwidge Danticat is the author of two novels, *Breath, Eyes, Memory,* and *The Farming of Bones,* and a collection of short stories, *Krik? Krak!,* which was nominated for the National Book Award in 1995. She is also the editor of *The Beacon Best of 2000: Great Writing by Women and Men of All Colors.*

Sandy Alexandre was born and raised in Brooklyn, New York and is a graduate of Dartmouth College. She is currently pursuing a doctorate in English at the University of Virginia.

Patricia Benoît is a filmmaker living in New York City.

Jean-Pierre Benoît is Professor of Economics and Law at New York University.

Martine Bury is a freelance writer. Her work has appeared in several publications including *Vibe, Jane, Nylon,* and *The Source.*

Jean-Robert Cadet holds a master's degree in French literature and teaches French and American history in Cincinnati, Ohio. *Restavec: From Haitian Slave Child to Middle-Class American* is his first book.

Anthony Calypso is an actor who writes both fiction and nonfiction. He is a graduate of the MFA program in fiction at Sarah Lawrence College. He is at work on his first novel.

Sophia Cantave is a doctoral candidate in American literature and a lecturer at Tufts University. She is the author of an essay "Who Gets to Create Lasting Images? The Problem of Black Representation in *Uncle Tom's Cabin*," in *Approaches to Teaching Stowe's Uncle Tom's Cabin*. She is also author of "Geography, Language, and Hyphens: Felix Morrisseau-Leroy and a Changing Haitian Aesthetic," published in *The Journal of Haitian Studies*.

Leslie Casimir is a journalist, currently working in New York City at the *Daily News*.

Myriam J. A. Chancy is the author of *Searching for Safe Spaces: Afro-Caribbean Women Writers in Exile* (Temple University Press, 1997) and *Framing Silence: Revolutionary Novels by Haitian Women* (Rutgers University Press, 1997). Currently residing in Phoenix, Arizona, she is associate professor of English at Arizona State University, Tempe. She is at work on a novel entitled *The Serpent's Claw* and on a literary memoir focusing on Haiti and the Latin Caribbean.

Leslie Chassagne, born in Haiti and raised in New York City since the age of nine, studied art and language in the New York City University system and is currently a teacher at the Young Adult

Learning Academy and Hunter College's International Language Institute. He is a poet, painter, and musician and has traveled throughout the Caribbean and Colombia.

Marc Christophe was born in Saint Marc, Haiti. He is professor of
French and Caribbean literature at Howard University. This excerpt
was adapted from his poem "PRESENT PASSE FUTUR" which
was published in his 1988 collection of poetry *Le Pain de L'Exile*
(The Bread of Exile).

Joel Dreyfuss is a former senior editor at *Fortune* and a regular con-
tributor to *The Haitian Times*.

Phebus Etienne is a poet living in Montclair, New Jersey.

Annie Grégoire is a teacher and an aspiring children's book writer.
She teaches second grade at Cush Campus Schools, a private school
in Brooklyn, New York. Grégoire received a master's degree in
foreign language education at New York University, where she has
also done extensive research in cross-cultural studies and children's
literature.

Maude Heurtelou is a native of Haiti, where she completed high
school. She holds an undergraduate degree from the San Carlos Uni-
versity/INCAP in Guatemala and a master's degree in public health
education. She has written over sixteen nonfiction books in Haitian
Kreyòl and two novels, *Lafami Bonplezi* and *Sezisman*, which have
been translated into English. She and her husband, Féquiere Vilsaint,
are the founders and publishers of Educavision, a publishing company.

Joanne Hyppolite was born in Haiti. Her family settled in the United States when she was four years old and she grew up in Boston. She has published two popular children's books, *Seth and Samona* (Delacorte Press, 1995), which won the Marguerite DeAngell Prize for New Children's Fiction and *Ola Shakes It Up* (Delacorte, 1998). Her fiction addresses the Haitian-American experience.

Dany Laferrière was born in Haiti, where he practiced journalism under Duvalier. He went into exile in Canada in 1978; soon after, he began working on his first novel *How to Make Love to a Negro*, which became an instant bestseller in both the original French and in English and was made into a feature film. He now divides his time between Montreal and Miami.

Marie-Hélène Laforest currently makes her home in Italy, where she teaches postcolonial literatures at the Instituto Universitario Orientale, Naples.

Francie Latour is a journalist, currently working at *The Boston Globe*.

Danielle Legros Georges is a writer living in Boston. Her work has been anthologized in *The Beacon Best of 1999*.

Miriam Neptune, age twenty-three, was born in the United States and raised in Los Angeles. She has taken an active interest in Haiti/ U.S. relations since the start of the 1991 coup, and hopes to produce documentary work on this subject. She is now a graduate student in New York University's Media and Culture program.

Nikòl Payen received her B.A. in journalism from SUNY New Paltz and her MFA in creative nonfiction from Sarah Lawrence College.

She was an assistant editor at *Essence Magazine*, where her writing has been featured. Other publications where her work has appeared include *The Daily News Caribbeat, The Crab Orchard Review, Third World Viewpoint, New World*, and a host of newsletters. Currently she is a professor of public speaking at Kingsborough Community College and is working on her forthcoming book, *Something in the Water*.

Marilene Phipps is a painter and poet. Author of *Crossroads and Unholy Water*, a collection of poetry published by Southern Illinois University Press, she is the winner of *The Crab Orchard Review* Poetry Prize and the Grolier Poetry Prize. She has won fellowships from the Guggenheim Foundation, Harvard's Bunting Institute, and the Harvard Center for the Study of World Religions. Her paintings have been exhibited in gallery and museum shows in Haiti, the United States, and throughout the world.

Garry Pierre-Pierre is the publisher and founder of *The Haitian Times*. He has worked as a reporter for *The New York Times* and *The Sun Sentinel*.

Marie Nadine Pierre is currently living in Miami, Florida. She is a doctoral candidate in the Comparative Sociology Department at Florida International University. Her dissertation will examine issues of body, foods, and dress for Haitian women in the Miami area.

Assotto Saint, (né Yves Lubin) was born in Haiti in 1957. He moved to New York in 1970 and was a performer with the Martha Graham Dance Company for many years. His *nom de guerre*, Assotto Saint, is derived from the combination of the name of a *Vodou* drum and that of Haitian Independence leader Toussaint Louverture, one of his heroes. An AIDS activist, he died in 1994, when he was thirty-seven years old.

Barbara Sanon is a Haitian-American filmmaker living in New York City.

Patrick Sylvain was born in Port-au-Prince Haiti and immigrated to the United States in 1981. He works as a bilingual education teacher in Massachusetts. His work has appeared in several literary magazines, including *Callaloo, The Caribbean Writer, Compost, Agni,* and *Ploughshares* as well as in the anthology *The Beacon Best of 1999.* He is the author of several books of poetry in Haitian *Kreyòl,* including *Mazakwa, Zanzèt,* and *Twokèt Lavi.*

Marie Ketsia Théodore-Pharel, born in Haiti, currently lives in Jupiter, Florida, with her infant daughter and husband and teaches at West Palm Beach Community College. *I'll Fly Away,* her first picture book, was published in 1999 by Educavision Publishing Company. Her short stories have been published in magazines. "The Mango Tree" appeared in *Compost* magazine in 1994; "Soup Joumou: Diary of a Mad Woman," in 1996; and "Light Chocolate Child," in *African Homefront* in 1995.

Michel-Rolph Trouillot is the author *of Peasants and Capital: Dominion in the World Economy* and *Haiti, State Against Nation: The Origins and Legacy of Duvalierism.* "Looking for Columbus" is the epilogue from his book *Silencing the Past: Power and the Production of History,* published by Beacon Press in 1996.

Gina Ulysse was born in Haiti in 1966. When she was twelve, her family migrated to the East Coast of the United States. In 1991, she earned a B.A. in English and Anthropology at Upsala College in New Jersey. She received her Ph.D. in Anthropology from the University of Michigan in 1999. She is currently assistant professor of African-American Studies at Bates College in Lewiston, Maine, as well as a committed social activist and spoken-word artist.

Katia Ulysse lives in Washington, D.C. "Mashe Petyon" is part of a book manuscript inspired by her collection of Haitian art.

Babette Wainwright is a licensed psychotherapist and a painter. She has lived in Madison, Wisconsin, since 1985.

🌹 GLOSSARY

Aba Duvalier   Down with Duvalier!

akra   malanga fritter (malanga: edible root)

andeyò/peyi andeyò   the Haitian provinces, the countryside, home of the Haitian peasantry

bal   dance party

bannann peze   sliced and pressed fried plantains

blan   white person, but also used to refer to foreigners in general

bonnanj   soul, basic life source

Bouki/Malis   opposite characters in Haitian folktales–(Bouki the fool and Malis the shrewd)

Bwa chèch   dry wood, also used as a reply in riddles to the interjection (Tim, tim!)

boulèt   meatballs

diri kole   rice and beans cooked together

djondjon   black mushrooms primarily used in a rice dish

dous   sweet confection, often with the consistency of fudge

egare   lost, dumb, confused

granmè   grandmother

griyo   fried pork

gwayabèl   light embroidered shirt worn primarily by men

kremas   a sweet coconut and milk-based liqueur

kenèp   Spanish limes

ki jan ou ye?   how are you?

kivèt   washbasin

kolon   colonist

konpè   friend, pal, also godfather of someone's child

konpa   variety of modern popular dance music

kouzen   cousin

l ap mòde ou   It will bite you

lavil   the city, downtown

leve mò   raising the dead

lougawou   woman who is human by day and vampire by night

lwa   spirit of the *Vodou* religion

madansara   tradeswoman, vendor, merchant

manman   mother

mapou   large tree with magic powers according to popular belief

marenn   godmother

marasa   twins, also *Vodou* spirit

matant   aunt

matinèt   a whip constructed with a piece of wood at the end of which are attached thin leather strips

mayi moulen   cornmeal dish

mesye sara   a male variation of madansara. Not very commonly used, but used here to indicate that some males now do participate in the intricate trade and travel network of local and international madansaras

mèsi   thank you

mizik rasin   modern music influenced by *Vodou* and *rara*

monnonk   uncle

moun   person, human being

m pa pi mal   I am fine, literally "not doing so bad"

mwen menm   I, as for myself, as far as I am concerned

parenn   godfather

pen patat   sweet potato-based desert

peristil   place of worship in *Vodou*

pikliz   a hot relish often made with hot peppers, chopped cabbage, vegetables and vinegar

pwa   beans

rara   an informal musical band parading

restavèk   unpaid child servant often treated as the slaves were in colonial time

san manman   motherless, used pejoratively to insult someone displaying bad behavior

tchaka   dish of cornmeal with beans and meat

ti   little, often used before someone's name to form a nickname

Tim, tim!   interjection used before posing a riddle

vagabon   rascal, shameless person

vaksin   musical instrument made out of bamboo reed

vèvè   ritual design traced on ground of *Vodou* worship places to invoke a specific spirit

Yanvalou   dance or *Vodou* rhythm

French Words

certificat   state exam at the end of elementary school

gourde   Haitian currency

Griots   storytellers in West Africa

gendarme   policeman, a member of the Haitian Army until 1995